HIV and AIDS

Oxfam GB

Oxfam GB, founded in 1942, is a development, humanitarian, and campaigning agency dedicated to finding lasting solutions to poverty and suffering around the world. Oxfam believes that every human being is entitled to a life of dignity and opportunity, and it works with others worldwide to make this become a reality.

Oxfam GB is a member of Oxfam International, a confederation of 13 agencies of diverse cultures and languages, which share a commitment to working for an end to injustice and poverty – both in long-term development work and at times of crisis.

For further information about Oxfam's publishing, and online ordering, visit www.oxfam.org.uk/publications

For information about Oxfam's development, advocacy, and humanitarian relief work around the world, visit www.oxfam.org.uk

HIV and AIDS

Edited by Alice Welbourn with Joanna Hoare

Oxfam

Practical Action Publishing Ltd
25 Albert Street, Rugby, CV21 2SD, Warwickshire, UK
www.practicalactionpublishing.com

First published by Oxfam GB in 2008.
Reprinted by Practical Action Publishing

This edition © Oxfam GB 2008

Oxfam GB is registered as a charity in England and Wales (no. 202918) and Scotland
(SCO 039042).
Oxfam GB is a member of Oxfam International.

Paperback ISBN: 978-0-85598-603-2
PDF ISBN: 9780855987671
Book DOI: https://doi.org/10.3362/9780855987671

A catalogue record for this publication is available from the British Library.

Cover photo: Participants at a workshop for teenagers on HIV and AIDS awareness,
Port au Prince, Haiti, 2007 (Caroline Irby/Oxfam)

Reasonable efforts have been made to publish reliable data and information, but the
author and publisher cannot assume responsibility for the validity of all materials or for
the consequences of their use.

The manufacturer's authorised representative in the EU for product safety is
Lightning Source France, 1 Av. Johannes Gutenberg, 78310 Maurepas, France.
compliance@lightningsource.fr

Working in Gender and Development

The *Working in Gender and Development* book series brings together themed selections of the best articles from the journal *Gender & Development* and other Oxfam publications, repackaged in book form to reach a wide audience of development practitioners and policy makers, and students and academics. Titles in this series present the theory and practice of gender-oriented development in a way that records experience, describes good practice, and shares information about resources. As such, they will contribute to and review current thinking on the gender dimensions of particular development and relief issues.

Other titles in the series include:
    Gender-Based Violence

Acknowledgements

All materials in this book other than those listed below are copyright © Oxfam GB 2008. The following items, which have been previously published as indicated, are copyrighted as shown.

'HIV/AIDS, globalisation, and the international women's movement' (pages 3–8) by Sisonke Msimang, first published in *Gender & Development* Volume 11, Number 1, March 2003, copyright © Oxfam GB 2003.

'Challenges and opportunities for promoting the girl child's rights in the face of HIV/AIDS' (pages 9–19) by Mildred Tambudzai Mushunje, first published in *Gender & Development* Volume 14, Number 1, March 2006, copyright © Oxfam GB 2006.

"I'm too young to die': HIV, masculinity, danger, and desire in urban South Africa' (pages 20–31) by Shannon Walsh and Claudia Mitchell, first published in *Gender & Development* Volume 14, Number 1, March 2006, copyright © Oxfam GB 2006.

'A gendered response to HIV/AIDS in South Asia and the Pacific: insights from the pandemic in Africa' (pages 32–43) by Madhu Bala Nath, first published in *Gender & Development* Volume 14, Number 1, March 2006, copyright © Oxfam GB 2006.

'Safe motherhood in the time of AIDS: the illusion of reproductive 'choice'' (pages 44–57) by Carolyn Baylies, first published in *Gender & Development* Volume 9, Number 2, July 2001, copyright © Oxfam GB 2001.

'Diversifying gender: male to female transgender identities and HIV/AIDS programming in Phnom Penh, Cambodia' (pages 61–74) by Barbara Earth, first published in *Gender & Development* Volume 14, Number 2, July 2006, copyright © Oxfam GB 2006.

'HIV-positive African women surviving in London: report of a qualitative study' (pages 92–101) by Lesley Doyal and Jane Anderson, first published in *Gender & Development* Volume 14, Number 1, March 2006, copyright © Oxfam GB 2006.

'Mitigating impacts of HIV/AIDS on rural livelihoods: NGO experiences in sub-Saharan Africa' (pages 105–22) by Joanna White and John Morton, first published in *Development in Practice* Volume 15, Number 2, March 2005, copyright © Oxfam GB 2005.

'Danger and opportunity: responding to HIV with vision' (pages 123–36) by Kate Butcher and Alice Welbourn, first published in *Gender & Development* Volume 9, Number 2, July 2001, copyright © Oxfam GB 2001.

Contents

List of Contributors

Jane Anderson is Director of the Centre for Study of Sexual Health and HIV, Homerton University Hospital NHS Foundation Trust, London.

Madhu Bala Nath has worked on gender, HIV, and AIDS for UNIFEM, UNDP, and UNAIDS. She is currently Regional Director for the South Asia Regional Office of the International Planned Parenthood Federation.

Carolyn Baylies was Reader in the Sociology of Developing Countries in the School of Sociology & Social Policy at the University of Leeds when she died in November 2003. She carried out influential research on the social impact of HIV and AIDS in Africa. Publications such as *AIDS, Sexuality and Gender in Africa*, produced jointly with Dr Janet Bujra and the Gender and AIDS Group in Zambia and Tanzania brought her international renown.

Kate Butcher has worked in HIV since the late 1980s. She is currently an independent consultant working as HIV mainstreaming advisor for AusAID's Papua New Guinea programme. She is also a regular consultant to Irish Aid, providing technical advice on a range of HIV-related issues, and practical guidance on addressing gender inequalities and HIV in development work. Kate is also on the board of the International Community of Women Living with HIV/AIDS.

Lesley Doyal is a Professor at the School for Policy Studies, University of Bristol.

Barbara Earth is an independent scholar based in Honolulu, Hawaii, where she is studying American Sign Language. She has experience in gender, HIV, and AIDS research in both Africa and Asia.

Joanna Hoare was Acting Editor on *Gender & Development* journal between July 2006 and June 2007. She is now working towards a Ph.D in the Department of Development Studies at the School of Oriental and African Studies, University of London.

The International Community of Women Living with HIV/AIDS (ICW) is the only international network of HIV-positive women. Members work with local, national, and international networks, organisations, and groups supporting and campaigning for the rights of HIV-positive women and men.

Claudia Mitchell is a James McGill Professor in the Faculty of Integrated Studies in Education at McGill University. Her research areas focus on visual methodologies, youth, gender and HIV and AIDS, gender-based violence in education, girlhood and popular culture, and teachers' self-study.

John Morton is Professor in Development Anthropology and Associate Research Director of the Natural Resources Institute, University of Greenwich, London.

Sisonke Msimang is Programme Director of the Open Society Initiative for Southern Africa (OSISA), where she also serves as the Manager of the HIV and AIDS Programme. For the last decade, she has worked on HIV, sexual and reproductive health, and women's rights with a range of NGOs and international agencies across Southern Africa.

Mildred T. Mushunje is a Senior Programme Manager with Catholic Relief Services (Zimbabwe), responsible for gender and child protection. She is also a Ph.D. candidate (Kellogg Fellow) in Social Policy; her thesis focuses on child-headed households and food security.

Janet Seeley is a Senior Lecturer in Gender and Development at the School of Development Studies, University of East Anglia. She provided advice on mainstreaming gender and HIV and AIDS in the programme of Australian support to Papua New Guinea's (PNG) National Agricultural Research and Development Agencies, and in the PNG Infrastructure Sector's intervention under the Transport Sector Support Programme. Since early 2007 Janet has been providing similar advice in the implementation of the Australian-funded 'Agricultural Research and Development Support Facility' in PNG.

Shannon Walsh is a researcher, filmmaker, and social activist currently working towards her Ph.D. in education and anthropology at McGill University.

Alice Welbourn is a writer, trainer, and activist with 30 years' experience in gender, health, HIV, and international community development. She wrote 'Stepping Stones', a training programme on relationship skills; she advises the United Nations and NGOs; and she formerly chaired The International Community of Women Living with HIV/AIDS (ICW).

Joanna White is an independent development consultant currently based in Hanoi, Viet Nam.

Introduction

Alice Welbourn

Overview

HIV (the Human Immunodeficiency Virus) and AIDS (Acquired Immune Deficiency Syndrome; the syndrome that can develop as a result of the virus' effects on the body[1]) have now been around for 25 years. This is almost the same number of years as the current life expectancy in some of the countries where there is the highest prevalence of HIV. The effect of AIDS has reduced life expectancy in these countries to as little as 33 years (UNICEF 2005).[2] All countries in the world have been affected by HIV and AIDS in some way.

As a biological virus, HIV is so successful because the conditions for its development and spread have been in existence for thousands of years. These include the universal power imbalances and conflicts produced by the following: sexism, racism, homophobia, ageism, the attitudes and practices of the rich world towards the majority world, religious and cultural imperialism, and taboos around sex, disease, sickness, and death. HIV is like the most invasive of all weeds, suffocating all in its path, since the conditions for its growth and spread are so deeply rooted in the injustices facing those who are poorest, most marginalised, and most voiceless in all our societies. These conditions and taboos are social, economic, and political in nature, affecting the development of all of us, wherever we live. They reach to the core of all our belief systems. If we wish to curb the spread of HIV effectively and in a sustainable way, it follows that it is these conditions, the root causes of HIV, which need to be challenged and changed. *Without* addressing the global causes, we will not only be unable to mitigate the global effects of HIV and AIDS, we will also be unable to achieve the Millennium Development Goals by the beginning of the 22nd century, let alone by 2015 (Hecht *et al.* 2006).

The world's major institutions have all paid attention to the enormity of the HIV and AIDS threat, to a greater or lesser degree. But all of them are failing to understand the roots of the problem – namely the inherent conditions listed above which are driving the pandemic. In particular, there is an institutional refusal to accept or address the fact that gender inequality is fuelling the spread of HIV throughout the world. For instance, the Global Fund to fight AIDS, Tuberculosis and Malaria (GFATM) has a large budget, a low-cost administrative approach, is relatively transparent, has fast funding mechanisms, and is ideally placed to lead the major responses to HIV in most countries through its Country Coordinating Mechanisms (CCM).[3] However, these responses are compromised by a consistent failure to consult and include women (particularly HIV-positive women) and women's civil-society organisations, and by the absence of a gendered monitoring mechanism to assess how its interventions impact on women and men.

Elsewhere, in certain cases, the activities of major institutions are worsening the effects of the pandemic. The US government's 'President's Emergency Programme for AIDS Response' (PEPFAR) is the world's largest single donor to HIV and AIDS programmes,[4] but only focuses on a limited number of key priority countries, and is currently constrained by a conservative approach to HIV prevention. This approach, based on right-wing fundamentalist Christian values, and not on a clear and widely documented scientific evidence-base (especially in relation to prevention messages, harm reduction, and access to condoms) has caused the disruption and collapse of many sound programmes in PEPFAR-funded countries. The influence of the International Monetary Fund's structural adjustment policies (SAPs) on public-sector wage bills has led to excessively low wage-ceilings in many of the countries most directly hit by HIV and AIDS, resulting in fewer staff in the education and health sectors (Marphatia *et al.* 2007). Shortages in both these sectors have negative, long-term effects on the capacities of these countries to respond to the HIV and AIDS crisis, and in particular on their capacities to support women and girls in both prevention and treatment programmes.

This collection of articles, drawn largely from Oxfam's journal *Gender & Development*, starts out by highlighting the role of many of these social, economic, and political conditions in generating the challenges which cause us all to be affected by HIV and AIDS. It then moves on to describe several of the more positive, largely community-based responses in different parts of the world. It is designed to be read by development and humanitarian practitioners and policy makers (be they gender specialists or others who are nonetheless interested in how gender connects to HIV and their work), and by academics and students concerned with HIV as a human-rights and development issue.

The collection is best read in conjunction with the first volume in this series, which focused on gender-based violence. Many of the issues addressed in that volume correspond closely to the issues raised by gender and HIV. It is recognised that gender violence is both a cause and a consequence of HIV and AIDS throughout the world (UNAIDS 2006; ICW and GCWA n.d.).[5] It is also clear that HIV, like gender-based violence, is a human-rights, a development, a public-health, and a humanitarian issue. Readers will also see an overlap in many of the themes raised by both volumes, which are as relevant to responses to HIV as they are to responses to gender-based violence. These themes include lack of political will to acknowledge the role of gender inequities in shaping all our lives; lack of appropriate legislation or changes in attitude; the need for changes in behaviours negotiated through discussions at the *local* level; the need for male involvement in both analysis of the issues, and in the development of new solutions; and the importance of supporting women's agency as activists and not just as victims. Both volumes also call for a holistic, multi-dimensional response to the issues in question.

This collection seeks to raise awareness about the enormity of the impact of gender inequalities, HIV, and AIDS on our lives and our work as development practitioners, while giving hope and suggestions for practical action to its readers. Readers from countries where there is a high prevalence of HIV will already have lost many friends, relatives, and colleagues to HIV. It is often hard for those of us living in the West, where we have largely been safe from armed conflict, and are too young to remember the Second World War, to appreciate the huge effect of the burden of grief that multiple bereavements cause. Thus we are often in danger of writing in ways which over-simplify, or just forget the effects of such chronic stress on the simplest of daily activities for those most deeply affected. HIV presents particular challenges because it still produces a grief which most of those experiencing it dare not share with others, for fear of isolation or hostility from friends, family, and colleagues, and even job loss. Non-government organisations (NGOs) are now far better than they used to be at supporting staff who, for instance, have experienced chronic stress and trauma in their work in conflict zones. But HIV, and gender inequities, their causes and consequences, are still subjects which – like gender violence – are deeply taboo and hidden away from friends and colleagues, even in countries where they are most prevalent. Carrying that inner burden of grief, without being able to name or share it properly with friends, colleagues, fellow members of a faith group, or other family members, is an especially draining kind of pain which few of us yet fully appreciate.

No quick fixes

If there is one thing which is clear about the links between gender and HIV, it is that they are *not* simple. Rather, they are made up of many complex and interwoven psychosocial, economic, legal, political, historical, and religious factors. Trying to compile a 200-page book that covers them all is a nigh impossible task. HIV, like gender, just can't be fitted into neat boxes.

This collection is therefore a personal response to these issues, based on my own personal perspectives and experiences over the past 25 years of my working life.

I was an Oxfam development worker – a deputy country representative – in the late 1980s, and I have been HIV-positive for about 18 years now. Before I became HIV positive, I worked on gender, health, and community-development issues with staff in a programme in East Africa. HIV was then just newly emerging. I could see that both national and international colleagues faced sexual and reproductive health issues and problems that did not have simple solutions. When information about HIV began to emerge, I sought to raise my own awareness of HIV, and the awareness of my colleagues, both those working for Oxfam, and those working for other agencies. However, I was told by managers from Oxfam and other agencies that it was not the role of an NGO to become involved in people's personal lives in that way. Soon afterwards, I did some consultancy work for another NGO, for which I drew up a preparatory paper to study quality of life issues affecting communities where that agency worked. I proposed that the NGO might address three key areas of people's lives – physical, material, and psychological well-being. It was fortunate that my contract was already signed, because at that point the director of that NGO declared that I was not the right person for the job since, in his view, psychological well-being had nothing to do with development work.

These stories are not intended to point the finger at individual agencies. I think all British-based agencies, at least, in the late 1980s, would have responded in similar ways. But these stories reflect how much the world of development has had to confront new realities over the last 20 years, largely in the face of growing awareness of major issues such as gender violence, the use of rape and sexual violence as a weapon of war and of genocide,[6] and the devastating impact of HIV and AIDS.

For many in the NGO world at least, HIV is now firmly recognised as a development issue, affecting all aspects of an agency's work. However, owing perhaps to the nature of HIV as a communicable disease and a desire to find a 'quick fix', most responses to date have focused more on trying to treat HIV and AIDS as conditions which can be eradicated through the use of traditional public-health messages and controls. But HIV, even more than any other communicable disease, cannot be stopped using such narrow medical responses. Indeed, attempts to do so have enabled it to take root even more effectively in new populations. So for instance in the UK young men and women still do not think that HIV has anything to do with their lives, despite the fact that the UK has the highest rate of teenage pregnancies in Europe, high rates of human papilloma virus and chlamydia among teenagers, high rates of excessive alcohol use among young people, and high rates of domestic violence.[7] Accepting that HIV is not just a narrow health issue has helped the development sector to realise that in the context of HIV, there needs to be a change in conventional thinking around traditional, vertical approaches to development. The UN, civil society, governments, business, and faith-based organisations alike are slowly beginning to recognise the urgent need for a holistic response, where bridges are built and links forged between disciplines and institutions.

Personal as well as professional issues

For the most part, as development practitioners we are residentially, economically, and educationally quite separated from the 'beneficiaries' with whom we work. Because of our relatively privileged position, we may well find ourselves shocked and embarrassed to be personally affected by many of the issues related to gender roles and relations, as well as to HIV, raised in this collection. These might include what to do about an unhappy relationship, anxieties and arguments about how to pay the endless family bills this month, concerns about unwanted sexual advances from a work colleague or boss and who to tell who won't laugh at you, uncertainties about how to access good confidential information and support about an awkward health problem, how to reason effectively with your teenage son who is staying out late when you are absent on field trips, worries about getting pregnant again, fears about having to take time off to look after a sick family member who refuses to go to the doctor, questions from your boss about why you were late for work yet again. These issues may well keep us awake worrying at night and affect our ability to work or cope with daily chores. These are the very issues at the core of gender roles in our societies – who is expected to do what in our daily lives, and by whom. When we have crises of multiple family sickness and deaths to cope with as well, and don't feel able to talk about the root causes, the chronic stress can be overwhelming.

The issues listed above are also at the core of the spread of HIV – issues which normally go unmentioned in the formal arena of our working lives. When we trained as health staff, agricultural extensionalists, water engineers, teachers, or community-development workers, we were given clear practical challenges to face, and clear technical solutions to address them. If a patient presented with certain symptoms, you worked out what they had, gave them the right treatment, and they would get better. If rainwater was scarce, you supported community members to dig a well, or to dig a rainwater catchment micro-environment around their trees, to maximise growth. You knew what to expect in the work and you felt confident and well-equipped by your training to deal with it. Things didn't always go to plan: maybe the woman didn't have enough money to pay for the treatment after the first month, or the young men were sent off to war and the women in the village could not lift the lid off the well to maintain it (both gender issues of course). But at least you were given a practical technical job to do, and you got on with it, fairly confident that you were doing what you had been taught to do as well as you could, that you could discuss what had gone wrong with colleagues and community members, and think of a better way round the issue next time.

So to many it feels strange suddenly to be expected to deal with issues which we have not been trained to think about, let alone to address, and which we are also quietly grappling with in our own lives. Suddenly the development world can feel quite a different and uncertain place. But the world we live in has changed irreparably, owing to the enormity of the HIV pandemic, and all of us now need to support one another to address the prospect of this issue in our own lives, as well as in the lives of those with whom we work. Institutions also need to reflect on their own roles in offering support to their staff, as well as reflecting on their own – largely inadvertent – contribution to the spread of the pandemic through their actions.

Our view of 'others'

Individually and collectively we also need to consider how we relate to and treat 'others' in our lives, including and especially people with HIV.[8] To date it has been a natural reaction around the world, in the face of the enormity of people's fear, to assume that someone else is 'to blame' for HIV and that it is not 'my' problem. Instead, it is seen as a problem created and spread by 'loose' women, by 'immigrants', by 'gays', by people from the neighbouring country…by anyone but 'people like me'. These assumptions are frequently accompanied by the idea that those with HIV must somehow be to blame for having acquired the virus. This response, whilst widespread, has never been safe, valid, or just. As more information emerges about how HIV has touched all strata of society – rich and poor, educated and uneducated, male and female, within and outside marriage – around the whole world, there is now a need more than ever for each one of us to examine how we too can be the unwitting cause of the spread of HIV and the stigma which fuels it in the communities in which we work, and how HIV can also affect our own lives.

In several parts of the world, marriage, especially early marriage, is a risk factor for women for HIV acquisition (UNAIDS 2007). This means that rather than marriage protecting women, as has long been thought the case, women who are married are contracting HIV from their husbands, because they are unable to negotiate condom use or are coerced into having sex against their will. This means that they can be at *more* risk of contracting the virus than if they were single, or belonged to a supposed 'high-risk' group such as sex workers (GCWA 2004). Female staff in a Kenyan health centre said they saw no point in taking medicine to stop them getting HIV after accidentally pricking themselves with used hypodermic needles in the clinic, because they were already at risk of HIV every night in their marriage beds (Silvester *et al.* 2005). The shape of HIV is constantly changing and our knowledge and attitudes need to change with it, if we want to protect ourselves and those we love, and if we want to support and nurture the lives of those of us who already have it or who are affected by it.

As products of our own societies, and since HIV is already so widespread in the world, we need also to reflect carefully upon how we view HIV and people with HIV in our *own* communities, wherever they may be. All people, whatever their medical condition, have human rights which need to be upheld. Furthermore, it is now widely recognised that the most effective way in which people begin to realise how HIV may affect their own lives is by meeting someone from their own circle who is living openly with HIV. The shock of realising that this person is HIV-positive yet looks totally normal, fit, and healthy (if they are still asymptomatic, or if they are on timely treatment) is hugely effective, suddenly transforming the 'other' into 'someone like me'. But such encounters will only happen if HIV-positive people can feel confident that they will be treated with love, respect, care, support, and solidarity if they reveal their HIV status. Otherwise, they will remain silent and it will be to the great unknown loss of those around them.[9]

HIV is a virus, not a punishment. Like the influenza epidemic of 1919, which killed more people than the First World War of 1914–1918, or the Black Death, which decimated the medieval population of Europe, diseases happen. It is people who judge others, not diseases. The great difference with HIV is that it is *far* less contagious than influenza, or plague. HIV *is* a virus which we can contain, if only we all work together in participatory ways to support one another to contain it. But HIV's routes of transmission, through unprotected sex, infected blood, unsterile injections, and lack of appropriate care during or after childbirth, connect it with the root taboo subjects in all our societies globally – gender inequities, sex, intimate bodily fluids, religious and traditional beliefs, and birth and death themselves. It is all the more important, then, that we all recognise that HIV doesn't just happen to 'others' – those we tend to dismiss, as a result of the prejudices that we learn as we grow up – and that we all realise that HIV can and does affect all sections of society, wherever we live in the world.

Themes of this volume

The themes covered in this reader are by no means comprehensive. I seek instead to explore certain areas which I feel have been less well-developed in much of the literature to date.

Part I, entitled 'Exploring the root causes of HIV', seeks to frame the book in a range of historical, political, economic, legal, and social contexts. This includes a recognition of the links between HIV and globalisation. The links with colonial power, apartheid, economic exploitation of the South by the North, migrant labour, political upheaval, and the resulting HIV explosion in Southern Africa, which Sisonke Msimang raises in the first chapter, are critical themes also common to the spread of HIV in many other parts of the world. A similar effect in India is highlighted in Madhu Bala Nath's chapter later in this section.

In sub-Saharan Africa, three-quarters of all those infected with HIV among 15–24-year-olds are young women, reflecting their biological, social, and economic vulnerability to infection (UNAIDS n.d.). Writing about Zimbabwe, Mildred Tambudzai Mushunje raises the challenges faced by girls in the context of a human-rights approach, framed by the Convention of the Rights of the Child (CRC) and the Convention on the Elimination of All Forms of Discrimination Against Women (CEDAW).[10] She rightly highlights the connections between these two conventions, something which is often forgotten by some more child-focused agencies, whose activities tend not to focus on keeping children's mothers alive and well and productive, despite this being what a child would like most. Mushunje discusses the multiple, chronic, physical, psychological, sexual, and material traumas facing girls with little or no personal autonomy within the broader political context of Zimbabwe today, where donor funds are frozen. Mushunje concludes with a strong list of practical actions which could support girls despite this challenging context. These suggestions can, and should, be widely replicated elsewhere.

Shannon Walsh and Claudia Mitchell's chapter on young men and violence in South Africa highlights how, once more, the current acceptance of violence amongst young men has grown out of the political, historical, and economic context. This chapter also reminds us clearly that gender is not just about women and girls, by illustrating how gender violence is also a risk factor for boys and young men. It is clear that in such contexts any fear of HIV is immaterial in the wider picture, and that risk-taking is expected. This chapter highlights our need to remember that we are all products of our gendered upbringings and that a simple 'boys are bad' analysis does not reflect well on any of us. The authors conclude by setting out real possibilities for change, whilst highlighting that unless and until current economic realities change, little else will.

Next, Madhu Bala Nath's chapter describes the different strands of HIV development in relation to gender in the Asia-Pacific region, proposing that there may be much to learn from Africa's experiences. This chapter provides a very useful overview analysis of the different reasons for the pandemic in this region, and indeed resonates closely with my understanding of what has happened in Africa.

The final chapter in this first section is Carolyn Baylies' piece on the illusion of reproductive 'choice' for women who may wish, or are pressured, to have children, but at the same time want to protect themselves and their children against HIV. For many women, wanting to become a mother is a biological urge, the strength of which is hard to describe. For many others, there is an added socially driven imperative, which dictates that they are not fully recognised by society as adults until they have given birth. Although Baylies draws mainly on her research in Zambia, and although the piece dates from 2001, the findings echo the experiences of HIV-positive women from many other countries and contexts, as documented in various publications by the International Community of Women living with HIV/AIDS (ICW). Women's fertility and sexual and reproductive rights – especially rights to motherhood – are especially affected by HIV status. Few women in many parts of the world have much access to decision-making over what happens to their bodies anyway, in terms of whom they marry, whether or not they have sex, when they have sex, and whether or not they have children. Once women are found to be HIV-positive – often from a test at an ante-natal clinic – these rights are even more eroded, as others dictate to them what they should do next with their lives. In Russia, when the women in one group of HIV-positive people wanted to talk about having children without risk of transmitting HIV to their babies, the men protested that they wanted to talk about 'serious' things and not 'women's' issues.[11]

Part II is entitled 'Rethinking 'our' attitudes to 'others'' realities'. Chapters in this section seek to raise awareness about 'others'' lifestyles, which may differ from our own. Thus they challenge the way in which we all assume that how we are or behave ourselves is 'good' and 'right', and how others are or behave is, by the very fact of its 'otherness', 'bad' and 'wrong'. This way of thinking tends to make us stand in judgement over people who may have different experiences of life from our own. Yet once we begin to learn more about their lives, from their own perspectives, it soon becomes clear that the story is more complex, and that our judgements are narrow and unjust, and borne out of our lack of knowledge or awareness of their lives. This section seeks to open up our minds to different realities by exploring the lives of sections of societies around the world, with whom many of us may be less familiar.

The first chapter in this section, by Barbara Earth, explores different gender identities in Cambodia. It stresses the inadequacy of the assumption that people are only male or female. It also challenges the widespread use of the term 'men who have sex with men' in many settings, since, as Earth points out, 'throughout time and place, there have been people whose bodies have not conformed to the two categories, "biological male" and "biological female".' Earth discusses the policy and programming implications of this to make HIV work meaningful and relevant to the groups concerned, and highlights how, ironically, the advent of HIV and AIDS 'may in fact be leading to new understandings not only of identity, but also of politics, community and agency'.

Then follows a newly commissioned piece on young men, expanding further on the risks to all of society, young men included, of perpetuating universal stereotypes which assume that in the context of sexual and reproductive rights, boys and their behaviour are somehow inherently bad. Examples are drawn from many different places, including research in Northern Europe and the USA, work with young men and women to address gender stereotypes in Eastern Europe, and other projects in India, Africa, Nicaragua, and Brazil that have successfully encouraged young men to reconsider their attitudes to sex. The authors highlight the sexual and reproductive health needs and rights of young men, and the huge global gap in services appropriate for them; the need to support young men in the way they view their male identities from early childhood, as a part of a life-long process of learning; and the particular issues facing young men who are HIV-positive, including those who are also fathers. The chapter emphasises the critical importance of involving young men – including young men with HIV – in any work related to HIV, in order that they may grow to see themselves, and to be seen, not as the problem but as valued members of society, who form an essential part of the solution to HIV prevention.

Lesley Doyal and Jane Anderson describe in their chapter the experiences of women who are HIV-positive Africans in the UK. The chapter explodes several racist myths popular in the British media – for instance that HIV-positive women are predominantly poor and uneducated, and come to the UK as 'health tourists'. The women interviewed had experienced multiple traumas, but showed immense resilience, despite their generally negative treatment by UK society.

In Part III, 'Practical multiple approaches', three chapters explore practical ways of addressing HIV and related issues. The authors point out both how HIV can affect many different sections of society and the economy, and how different interventions across a wide range of sectors can serve to reduce infections and mitigate the impact of HIV on communities. The first chapter, by Joanna White and John Morton, spells out the enormity of the AIDS disaster for livelihoods, knowledge inheritance, and the rural economy in sub-Saharan Africa. White and Morton describe the widespread effects of AIDS on development work in general, and emphasise the importance of innovative ways in which NGOs that have not previously addressed HIV can create initiatives which support people affected by AIDS. In particular, they discuss how women and young people can be supported, given that they are normally left out of agricultural extension or income-generating programmes, yet often become heads of households through AIDS-related sickness and death.

The second chapter, by Kate Butcher and myself, describes a variety of different programmes, from HIV-focused projects with sex workers in Bradford, the UK, and Nepal (for whom immediate fears of violence from clients and police, not HIV, was the main concern), to workshops with DFID national staff in Pakistan. The role of traditional healers and of research conducted by HIV-positive women themselves is also discussed. The chapter concludes by emphasising once more the need to include the people who are the focus of activities from the outset; the need to engage men as well as women; the need for a gender-aware response; and the need to plan ahead to work in these ways in countries where HIV prevalence is so far low, in order to keep it that way.

This section concludes with a chapter which describes efforts to do just this in Papua New Guinea, a country with one of the highest levels of gender violence in the world. Janet Seeley and Kate Butcher describe the innovative but simple ways adopted to mainstream HIV awareness and gender into the oil-palm industry, in order to promote women's economic independence and reduce conflict and gender-based violence.

Part IV focuses on 'Positive agency and action'. This section contains a chapter describing an advocacy training workshop run by and for HIV-positive women in Southern Africa (all of whom are members of ICW), on their sexual and reproductive rights. This chapter serves to remind us of the importance of considering HIV-positive women not just as 'victims' but as active agents of change (see McGovern 2006). It is a sad irony of this pandemic that ICW is the only international network run for and by HIV-positive women, with members from over 130 countries on every continent, but many still have not heard of it. The organisation has produced many publications on a wide range of issues relating to HIV-positive women's rights, based on research conducted by HIV-positive women themselves, but hardly any are cited by others writing about HIV and gender issues, despite their widespread availability through the Internet. This prompts us to consider the nature and validity of different forms of knowledge, since the lack of citation of HIV-positive people's work would suggest that their research is somehow considered less 'valid' than work conducted on them by others. This question will be discussed further in the conclusion.

All these chapters illustrate the role of gender norms in shaping our identities throughout our lives, a concept which often runs so deep that many still fail to recognise it, and deny its relevance, both to our lives, and to HIV.[12] The chapters also underline the fundamental importance of working with communities directly, in order to create a climate of hope, understanding, and ability to cope, rather than one of fear, threat, and hopelessness. In this way responses can draw from the humanity inherent in us all.

References

Dickson, A. (2003) *A Voice for Now: Changing the Way We See Ourselves as Women*, London: Piatkus Books.

Global Coalition on Women and AIDS (GCWA) (2004) 'HIV prevention and protection efforts are failing women and girls', press release, 2 February 2004, available at: http://data.unaids.org/Media/Press-Releases02/pr_gcwa_02feb04_en.pdf (last accessed September 2007).

Hecht, R., A. Alban, K. Taylor, S. Post, N.B. Andersen, et al. (2006) 'Putting It Together: AIDS and the Millennium Development Goals', PLoS Med 3(11), available at: http://medicine.plosjournals.org/archive/1549-1676/3/11/pdf/10.1371_journal.pmed.0030455-S.pdf (last accessed September 2007).

International Community of Women Living with HIV/AIDS (ICW) and the Global Coalition on Women and AIDS (GCWA) (n.d.) 'Violence against HIV positive women', London: ICW, available at: www.icw.org/files/VAW-ICW%20fact%20sheet-06.doc (last accessed September 2007).

McGovern, T. (2006) 'Models of resistance: 'victims lead'', *Health and Human Rights: an International Journal* 9 (2): 234–55.

Marphatia, A. A., R. Moussié, A. Ainger, and D. Archer (2007) 'Confronting the contradictions: the IMF, wage bill caps and the case for teachers', London: ActionAid, available at: www.actionaid.org/assets/pdf/AAConf_Contradictions_Final2.pdf (last accessed September 2007).

Silvester, L., J. Raven, J. Price, S. Theobald, I. Makwiza, S. Jones, N. Kilonzo, R. Tolhurst, M. Taegtmeyer, and G. Dockery (2005) 'Analysis of the gender dimension in the scale-up of antiretroviral therapy and the extent to which free treatment at point of delivery ensures equitable access for women', Liverpool: Gender and Health Group, Liverpool School of Tropical Medicine, Liverpool Associates in Tropical Health; Nairobi: Liverpool VCT, Care & Treatment; Lilongwe: Reach Trust, available at: www.liv.ac.uk/lstm/research/groups/documents/report_gender_equity_art_scale_up.pdf (last accessed September 2007).

UNAIDS (2006) 'Stop violence against women, fight AIDS', Geneva and Washington DC: UNAIDS, available at: http://womenandaids.unaids.org/themes/docs/UNAIDS%20VAW%20Brief.pdf (last accessed September 2007).

UNAIDS (2007) 'Statement to the Fifty-first session of the Commission on the Status of Women', 26 February–9 March 2007, New York: UNAIDS, available at: http://data.unaids.org/pub/Speech/2007/070302_csw_unaidsstatement.pdf (last accessed September 2007).

UNAIDS (n.d.) 'Women', Geneva and Washington DC: UNAIDS, available at: www.unaids.org/en/GetStarted/Women.asp (last accessed September 2007).

UNICEF (2005) 'HIV/AIDS: A deadly crisis each day in Zimbabwe', New York: UNICEF, available at: www.unicef.org/aids/zimbabwe_25834.html (last accessed September 2007).

Notes

1 Someone with HIV can carry the virus unknowingly for several years. When he or she starts to get sick regularly, owing to the effect of the virus on their body, or when their CD4 count (a measure of the strength of an individual's immune system: see www.aidsmap.com/cms1031944.asp, last accessed October 2007) reaches a low level, they are said to have AIDS. My CD4 count went down to under 200 in the year 2000, 11 years after I acquired HIV. So I then started on anti-retroviral treatment. My CD4 count is now 670 and I am fit and well and fully productive. If people with HIV are given the care, love, support, solidarity, respect, and the drugs they need, they can continue to live long and productive lives. This is why it is important for us all to talk about 'HIV and AIDS', rather than 'HIV/AIDS', in recognition that with the right response, an HIV diagnosis does not need to lead to rapid sickness and death. It should be noted, however, that many of the articles in this volume were first published in Oxfam's two journals before this distinction was made in Oxfam's house style.

2 In Botswana, half of all pregnant women aged 30–34 in 2005 were HIV-positive, and this figure is rising (AIDS Epidemic Update 2006, page 5, available at: http://data.unaids.org/pub/EpiReport/2006/04-Sub_Saharan_Africa_2006_EpiUpdate_eng.pdf). The largest growth in HIV in Western Europe is in the UK (see 'UNAIDS AIDS Epidemic Update 2006', page 56, available at: http://data.unaids.org/pub/EpiReport/2006/09North_America_Western_Central_Europe_2006_EpiUpdate_eng.pdf , last accessed September 2007). In the USA, four times as many African American women than from any other ethnic group die of HIV-related illness (see www.womancando.org/conditions/africanamerican.htm, last accessed September 2007).

3 For more information on the GFATM's Country Coordinating Mechanisms, please see www.theglobalfund.org/en/apply/mechanisms/ (last accessed September 2007).

4 www.whitehouse.gov/g8/2003/hivaids.html (last accessed September 2007).

5 See also interview with Purnima Mane, gender and HIV expert and current UNFPA Deputy Executive Director, available at: www.unaids.org/en/MediaCentre/PressMaterials/FeatureStory/2007030 8_Interview_Purnima_IWD2007.asp (last accessed September 2007).

6 For instance, the use of rape as a weapon of war in Rwanda led to high levels of HIV infection. See www.theforgivenessproject.com/stories/ mary-blewitt (last accessed September 2007).

7 www.womenandequalityunit.gov.uk/domestic_violence/key_facts.htm

8 For a fuller discussion on the ways in which we objectify others, see Dickson (2003).

9 To read some personal testimonies written by HIV-positive men and women, see: 'Fulfilling fatherhood: experiences from HIV positive fathers' (www.ippf.org/en/Resources/Reports-reviews/Fulfilling+Fatherhood. htm) and 'Dreams and desires: sexual and reproductive health experiences of HIV positive women' (www.ippf.org/en/Resources/Reports-reviews/ Dreams+and+Desires.htm), both published by the International Planned Parenthood Federation; 'Positive voices' – voices of women and men from faith-based communities who are members of the ANERELA network (www.stratshope.org/b-cc-01-positive.htm); and the website for 'UN+', the group for UN staff members who are openly HIV positive (www.unplus.org.). (All sites last accessed September 2007).

10 For a list of key rights instruments relevant to women and girls see www.icw.org/node/198 and www.worldywca.info/index.php/ywca/ world_council_iws/iws_women_s_summit/call_to_action/support_ documents_for_the_call_to_action (both last accessed September 2007).

11 Personal communication with Russian AIDS activist, June 2006.

12 See Dickson (2003) for a fuller discussion of this.

Part I
Exploring the root causes of HIV

1 HIV/AIDS, globalisation, and the international women's movement

Sisonke Msimang

HIV/AIDS and globalisation

Globalisation has been described as 'the drive towards an economic system dominated by supranational trade and banking institutions that are not accountable to democratic processes or national governments' (Globalisation Guide, www.globalisationguide.org /01.html). It is characterised by an increase in cross-border economic, social, and technological exchange under conditions of (extreme) capitalism. As human bodies move across borders in search of new economic and educational opportunities, or in search of lives free from political conflict and violence, they bring with them dreams and aspirations. Sometimes, they carry the virus that causes AIDS, and often, they meet the virus at their destinations.

As corporations increasingly patrol the planet, looking for new markets, and natural and human resources to exploit, they set up and abandon economic infrastructure – opening and closing factories, establishing hostels. In so doing, they create peripheral communities hoping to benefit from employment and the presence of new populations where previously there were none. And when they move on, once they have found a cheaper place to go, they leave in their wake communities that are extremely susceptible to HIV/AIDS.

This is because the virus follows vulnerability, crosses borders with ease, and finds itself at home where there is conflict, hunger, and poverty. The virus is particularly comfortable where wealth and poverty co-exist – it thrives on inequality. It is not surprising, then, that Southern Africa provides an excellent case study of the collusion between globalising processes and HIV/AIDS.

The economy of the region has been defined in the last two centuries by mining: gold and diamonds. In an era of plummeting gold prices, and an increasing shift towards the service industry, Southern Africa is shedding thousands of jobs. Yet the last century of globalisation has provided a solid platform for the current AIDS crisis.

3

If there was a recipe for creating an AIDS epidemic in Southern Africa, it would read as follows: 'Steal some land and subjugate its people. Take some men from rural areas and put them in hostels far away from home, in different countries if need be. Build excellent roads. Ensure that the communities surrounding the men are impoverished so that a ring of sex workers develops around each mining town. Add HIV. Now take some miners and send them home for holidays to their rural, uninfected wives. Add a few girlfriends in communities along the road home.

Add liberal amounts of patriarchy, both home-grown and of the colonial variety. Ensure that women have no right to determine the conditions under which sex will take place. Make sure that they have no access to credit, education, or any of the measures that would give them options to leave unhappy unions, or dream of lives in which men are not the centre of their activities. Shake well and watch an epidemic explode.'

There's an optional part of the recipe, which adds an extra spice to the pot: African countries on average spend four times more on debt servicing than they do on health. Throw in a bit of World Bank propaganda, some loans from the IMF, and beat well. Voilà. We have icing on the cake.

As the gap between the rich countries of the North and the poor countries of the South grows, we are beginning to see serious differences in the ways that states can afford to take care of their citizens. Access to technology, drugs, and strong social safety nets in the North, mean that HIV/AIDS is a manageable chronic illness in most developed countries. Yet there are pockets of poor, immigrant, gay, and otherwise marginalised communities within these countries, where HIV prevalence is on the rise. An analysis of the complex intersections between inequalities tells us that it is not enough to belong to a rich country – that alone does not protect you from vulnerability to HIV infection, nor does it guarantee treatment. Where you sit in relation to the state is equally important – whether you are a woman, a poor woman, a black woman, an educated woman, a lesbian, a woman with a disability who is assumed not to be having sex, an immigrant who is not entitled to many of the social security benefits of citizens. All these factors determine your vulnerability to HIV/AIDS.

Now what does this mean for a 25-year-old woman living in Soweto? Jabu works as a security guard at a shopping centre in Johannesburg. Every day she spends two hours travelling to work because of the distances the architects of apartheid set up between city centres and the townships that serviced them. Jabu is grateful to have a job. Her two little ones are in KwaZulu Natal with their grandmother until Jabu can get a stable job. She is on a month-to-month contract with the security company. She watches expensive cars all day, protecting their owners' investments while they work. The company doesn't want to take her on as staff so each month she faces the uncertainty of not having a job the next month. Joining a union is not an option – she's not technically a staff member and she can't afford to make trouble. Jabu's boyfriend Thabo drives a taxi. Their relationship saves her cash because he drives her to and from work every day – a saving of almost one-third of her salary each month. She has another boyfriend at work, who often buys her lunch. She has to be careful that Thabo doesn't find out.

In addition to race, class, and gender, Jabu's life is fundamentally shaped by the forces of globalisation – where she works and how secure that work is, where her children live, even how she arrives at work. These factors all influence her vulnerability to HIV infection.

HIV/AIDS and feminism

During the last eight years of my work on sexual and reproductive rights, my focus has been primarily on HIV and AIDS. For me, the pandemic brings into stark relief the fact that states have failed to provide their citizens with the basic rights enshrined in the declaration of human rights.

Twenty years ago, AIDS was known as Gay Related Immune Disease – so associated was it with gay men. Today, the face of AIDS has changed. It looks like mine. It is now black, female, and extremely young. In some parts of sub-Saharan Africa, girls aged 15–19 are six times more likely than their male counterparts to be HIV-positive. Something is very wrong.

In the next ten years, the epidemic will explode in Asia and in Central and Eastern Europe as well as in Latin America. The pandemic will have profound effects on the burden of reproductive work that women do, and this in turn will have far-reaching consequences for the participation of women in politics, the economic sector, and other sectors of society. The very maintenance of the household, the work that feminist economists like Marilyn Waring, Diane Elson, and others tell us keeps the world running, may no longer be possible.

As older women are increasingly called upon to care for children, and as life expectancy shrinks to the forties and fifties, in Africa we face the prospect of a generation without grandparents, and an imminent orphan and vulnerable children crisis that will effectively leave kids to take care of kids. As the orphan crisis deepens, child abuse is on the rise. Girls without families to protect them are engaging in survival sex to feed themselves and their siblings, and we are told that communities will 'cope.' There is a myth of coping that pervades the development discourse on AIDS. What it really means is that women will do it. What it translates into is that families split up, girls hook for money and food,[3] and a vicious circle is born.

While there is some feminist analysis of the AIDS epidemic, we have not yet heard a rallying cry from the women's movement. A recent article by Noeleen Heyzer, UNIFEM's Executive Director, begins to formulate some arguments about why in the context of AIDS, women can no longer wait for equality with men (www.csmonitor. com/2002/0718/p13s02-coop.html). Dr. Heyzer points out that it takes 24 buckets of water a day to care for a person living with AIDS – to clean sheets fouled by diarrhoea and vomit, to prepare water for bathing (sometimes several times a day), to wash dishes and prepare food. For women who must walk miles, and still do all the other chores that always need doing, the burden becomes unbearable.

This past spring in New York, I was asked to speak to a group at a high school in Brooklyn about HIV/AIDS and violence against women in the South African context. They were an intelligent group, well versed in feminism. I was not the only presenter. A young American woman who had worked with *Ms. Magazine* talked about pop culture, and the politics of wearing jeans and letting your G-string[4] show. I left the meeting feeling disconcerted. I had made my presentation and received a few awkward questions about men in Africa. I cringed on behalf of my brothers because I certainly was not trying to demonise them, but the students were feeding into a larger narrative of the familiar discourse of black male laziness, deviancy, and sexual aggression that I was careful to point out to them. Aside from that, they found little else to talk about.

On the other hand, the woman from the USA struck a chord with them. They talked about eating disorders and the media, about Britney Spears and Janet Jackson. It was fascinating. Having lived in the USA, I was able to follow and engage, but my interests as an African feminist do not lie in this subject matter. It was a clear example of how far apart we, as feminists, sometimes are from one another.

Contexts vary, and of course the issues that are central in the global North will be different from those of Southern feminists. And amongst us there will be differences. I understood where the high-school students were coming from. Indigenous feminism must be rooted in what matters most to women at a local level. At a global level within feminism, however, I fear that we may be in danger of replicating the G-strings versus AIDS conversation. I am worried by the relative silence from our Northern sisters about a pandemic that is claiming so many lives.

A way forward

In the context of HIV/AIDS, it is no longer enough to frame our conversations solely in terms of race, class, and gender. These are primary markers of identity, but increasingly, we need more. We need to look at where women are located spatially in relation to centres of political, social, and economic power. We need also to examine how where we live – rural, urban, North or South – intersects with poverty and gender. We also need to think about how the experience of poverty interacts with, and not just intersects with, gender. Culture is another factor that deserves attention.

We are beginning to see dangerous patriarchal responses to the epidemic – from virginity tests to decrees about female chastity from leaders. In part this is simply an extension of deeply rooted myths about female sexuality. However, with HIV/ AIDS, it can also be attributed to the fact that in many cases women are the first to receive news of their sero-positive status. This is often during pre-natal screening, or when babies are born sick. Bringing home the 'news' that there is HIV in the family often means being identified as the person who caused the infection in the first place. We know that, in the vast majority of cases, this is simply not true.

The Treatment Action Campaign (TAC), a movement begun by and for people living with HIV/AIDS in South Africa, has managed to mobilise national and international support for the idea of universal access to drugs for people with AIDS. The group began their campaign by using pregnant women as their rallying cry. The right to nevirapine for pregnant women opened the door for TAC's broader claims about the rights of all people with HIV/AIDS to HIV medication. The campaign has been hugely successful. TAC encouraged the South African government to take the pharmaceutical industry to court and the government won, paving the way for a win at the World Trade Organization. Companies' patent rights can no longer supersede the rights of human beings to access life-saving medicines.

TAC's strategy needs to be vigorously debated and analysed by feminists. TAC did not use arguments about reproductive and sexual rights. They simply said, 'It is unfair for the government not to give drugs to pregnant women so they can save their babies' lives.' It was a classic 'woman as the vessel' argument. TAC's interest was not in women's rights – but in the rights of people living with HIV/AIDS, some of whom happen to be women. The campaign's success was largely based on the notion that the average South African found it difficult to accept that 'innocent' babies would die because of government policy. This requires some serious feminist interrogation. TAC has since been pushed by gender activists within the movement to ensure that the drugs do not stop when the baby is born.

Gender activists to date have struggled to get their voices heard in the doctor-dominated AIDS world. The mainstream women's movement needs to get on board and face up to the challenge of HIV/AIDS. AWID's (The Association for Women's Rights in Development) 'Globalise This' campaign provides an opportunity to highlight the HIV/AIDS epidemic and the threat it poses to women.

At precisely the moment when we need international solidarity to focus on the impact of AIDS on poor women's lives, and their need to be able to control their lives and their bodies, we have to oppose the US administration's cutbacks on funding for essential reproductive health services. We are also still waiting for the G8 to enact their long-standing commitment to spend 0.7 per cent of GDP (gross domestic product) on overseas development assistance each year. How likely is it that they will ever reach this target if they focus instead on supporting the war against Iraq?

Our sisters in the North need to develop a consciousness about the fight against AIDS as a feminist fight. We need civil society and feminist voices in developing countries to challenge their governments to tackle HIV/AIDS as a health issue, as a human-rights issue, and as a sexual and reproductive rights issue. If we lose this fight, it will have profound effects on the lives of girls and women into the next century.

This article was originally published in Gender & Development, *volume 11, number 1, March 2003.*

Reference

Crenshaw Williams, K. (1994) 'Mapping the margins: intersectionality, identity politics, and violence against women of color', in M. Albertson Fineman and R. Mykitiuk (eds.) *The Public Nature of Private Violence*, New York: Routledge.

Notes

1 Treatment Action Campaign, a movement begun by and for people living with HIV/AIDS in South Africa, which began in the late 1990s.

2 I have based my idea of 'intersectionality' on Kimberlé Crenshaw's definition: for her, intersectionality is about 'challenging those groups that are home to us, in the name of those parts of ourselves that don't feel so at home' (Crenshaw Williams 1994).

3 Girls engage in survival sex/sexual relationships for financial gains.

4 Fashionable underwear.

2 Challenges and opportunities for promoting the girl child's rights in the face of HIV/AIDS

Mildred Tambudzai Mushunje

The nature and scope of childhood has dramatically changed in the context of the HIV/AIDS pandemic. A large proportion of children in Zimbabwe today do not experience true nurturing in their childhood. Their childhood is taking place against a backdrop of unprecedented political, economic, cultural, and social changes. Worst of all, the backdrop includes HIV/AIDS, the impact of which manifests itself in the breakdown of extended family safety nets, orphans' consequent loss of a protective family environment, and widespread child-headed households.

UNAIDS *et al.* (2004) estimates that globally, close to three million children under the age of 15 years have been infected with HIV. In 1996 alone, around 1,000 children died daily of AIDS and even more became infected. At the end of that year, it was estimated that 830,000 children under 15 years of age were living with the virus, a number that UNAIDS expected to rise to one million by the end of 1997. Well over 90 per cent of these children would be in developing countries.

In 2002, an estimated 1.8 million Zimbabweans were living with HIV/AIDS, of whom 240,000 were children. UNAIDS *et al.* (2004) reports that a third of the Zimbabwean population is HIV-positive, and a child dies every 15 minutes. Zimbabwe now has the fourth-highest number of people with HIV in the world, and life expectancy has declined from 61 years to only 33 years (UNICEF 2004). At the 2002 International AIDS Conference in Barcelona, UNAIDS projected that by 2005 Zimbabwe would have lost 19 per cent of its workforce to HIV/AIDS.

The Zimbabwe National Plan of Action (NPA) for Orphans and Vulnerable Children (OVC) estimates that there are currently 1.3 million orphans. Of these, about 980,000 have been orphaned by AIDS. In 2004 alone, 160,000 children lost a parent. The scale of the AIDS orphan crisis is somewhat masked by the time lag between HIV infection, death, and orphaning. Even if all new HIV infections were to stop today, the number of orphans would continue to rise for at least the next ten years (Fredriksson and Kanabus 2005). The impact of HIV/AIDS on children is catastrophic. Worst affected is the girl child.

Children's rights in the face of HIV/AIDS

The United Nations Convention on the Rights of the Child (CRC) provides a framework for promoting and protecting the rights of children, which can minimise the impact of the HIV/AIDS epidemic on them. Yet, despite its almost universal ratification, the response to infected, affected, and vulnerable children has remained inconsistent. Internationally, AIDS programmes for children have been ad hoc and fragmented and have lagged behind those for adults. As a consequence, children are faced with reduced protection, and are more vulnerable to neglect, abuse, and exploitation (UNICEF 1998).

The CRC, in the context of HIV/AIDS, has spelled out principles for reducing children's vulnerability to infection and for protecting children from discrimination because of their real or perceived HIV/AIDS status. Some of the provisions in the framework are as follows.

Children's right to life, survival and development should be guaranteed.

The civil rights and freedoms of children should be respected, with emphasis on removing policies that may result in children being separated from their parents or families.

Children should have access to HIV/AIDS prevention education, information and to the means of prevention. Measures should be taken to remove social, cultural, political or religious barriers that block children's access to these resources.

All children should receive adequate treatment and care for HIV/AIDS, including those children for whom this may entail additional costs because of their circumstances, such as orphans.

States should include HIV/AIDS as a disability, if disability laws exist, to strengthen the protection of people living with HIV/AIDS against discrimination.

Children should have access to health care services and programmes, and barriers to access encountered by especially vulnerable groups should be removed.

Children should have access to social benefits, including social security and social insurance.

Children should enjoy adequate standards of living.
(WHO 1995)

The Convention on the Elimination of All Forms of Discrimination Against Women (CEDAW) is complementary to the CRC, in as far as it protects the rights of the girl child. The convention obligates those countries that have ratified or acceded to it to take 'all appropriate measures' to ensure the full development and advancement of women in all spheres – political, educational, employment, health care, economic, social, legal, and marriage and family relations. It also calls for the modification of social and cultural patterns of conduct in order to eliminate prejudice, customs, and all other practices based on the idea of inferiority or superiority of either sex (Bennett-Haigney 2001).

At the national level, Zimbabwe has progressive child-protection instruments, the main one being the Children's Protection and Adoption Act (Children's Act). Other subsidiary instruments, including the National Plan of Action (2005) and the Orphan Care Policy (1999), promote the overall protection of the rights of the child. However, the crises that have enveloped Zimbabwe over the last few years have compromised the extent to which children can enjoy basic rights. Notwithstanding the challenges the nation currently faces, all member states who are signatory to the convention are obliged to ensure that the provisions within the convention are implemented. Children are the primary claimants of the CRC, and parents are the immediate duty bearers, who are responsible for the well-being of the child. Where the family is unable to exercise its obligations, the state should step in and reinforce support to the family. In Zimbabwe, the state enforces its protective role and oversight of children's rights through the Children's Act.

Challenges for the girl child in the face of HIV/AIDS

HIV/AIDS sets back development and changes patterns of life. To a child, this translates 'into a world turned upside down' (Guni 2005). Children do not need to have HIV/AIDS to be devastated by it (UNICEF 2004). When it enters a household, the very fabric of a child's life falls apart. Naturally, girls and boys are both affected by HIV/AIDS, but the effects and challenges are different. The next section discusses the challenges that the girl child faces. Despite the ratification of international instruments by the Zimbabwe government and the national legal framework for child protection, the rights of the girl child in the face of HIV/AIDS are greatly threatened.

Risks with HIV/AIDS in the family

When HIV/AIDS enters a family, even before the death of a parent, the girl child's life begins to take a downward tumble. This is encapsulated in the following: the mother falls sick, and therefore cannot do household chores; the eldest girl child becomes the one to take over the chores. As the mother falls ill, gets better and falls ill once more, the girl child will in turn be moving in and out of school. When the periods of illness grow longer as a parent moves towards death, the girl child will often also take extended time off from school to care for her parent. Parents with HIV also have to spend money on medication, and therefore some of the children are likely to be removed from school to save income. Often, it is the girl child or children who make way for their brothers to continue with school.

The failure to attend school also impacts on the girl's long-term health and survival. While both girls and boys are likely to drop out of school when they are orphaned, it is more likely that the girl child will be the first to drop out, to become the *de facto* head of household. A study in Zimbabwe based on household surveys involving more than 1,400 households with children under 16 found that 'the greater the number of years it is since a mother died the smaller the chance that a young girl will complete school' (Nyamukapa *et al.* 2003, 22).

The girl child loses out on her childhood, as she takes on an adult role. Other advantages associated with being in a protective school environment for the girl child are also lost. For most girls, education goes beyond learning, as a girl who is educated is in a better position to care for herself and less likely to fall prey to HIV. For most girls, it can be a lifesaver (UNICEF 2004). UNICEF (2004) also notes that even when orphaned girls do successfully enrol in school, their subsequent achievements may be lower because of persistent stereotypes and household responsibilities.

Increased vulnerability of orphans

Eventually, children suffer the death of their parent or parents, and the emotional trauma that results. The death of a parent means children are at risk of emotional deprivation and loss of affection, attention, and love, all of which can be emotionally damaging and traumatic. They experience grief and sorrow and may withdraw emotionally, a response that can have long-lasting, negative effects on their development. Some children whose parents have died as a result of AIDS may also be infected, and also need health care. Unfortunately, with limited resources at the family's disposal, many cannot afford basic health care and have little access to adequate food, thus increasing their vulnerability (UNICEF 2004).

The suffering of children is compounded, as the disease changes the family structure and exerts a heavy economic toll, often requiring children, particularly the girl children, to become both caretakers and breadwinners. Faced with economic hardships, girls become more vulnerable to prostitution, in which they have little power to negotiate for safe sex (UNICEF 2004). The loss of a parent also removes the protective factor that is contributory to securing children's rights. This further puts the girl child at risk of exploitation, both physical and emotional (Wakhweya *et al.* 2003), which may result in unwanted pregnancy, and possibly HIV or sexually transmitted infection. In adolescence, the risk of HIV infection increases rapidly and girls are more vulnerable (UNICEF 2004).

High levels of HIV/AIDS awareness among adolescents have not necessarily translated into behaviour change, and risk-taking continues to be common practice.

There are a number of factors that account for this. These include cultural and traditional attitudes and practices, economic vulnerability, unequal gender relations, issues of self-identity, knowledge and understanding of sexuality and HIV/AIDS, perceptions of one's own risk, and early sexual debut. There may be increased risk of being abused by men (such as male teachers or close male relatives) who hold greater economic and social power. Being isolated, girls are often threatened, and sworn to eternal silence.

Stigmatisation

Individual households struck by AIDS often suffer disproportionately from stigma, isolation, and impoverishment, and the emotional toll on the children is heavy. The impact is most acute on girls, already facing hardship or neglect. Children grieving for dying or dead parents may be stigmatised by society because of their association with HIV/AIDS. The distress and social isolation experienced by these children, both before and after the death of their parent(s), are strongly exacerbated by the shame, fear, and rejection that often surrounds people affected by HIV/AIDS (International HIV/AIDS Alliance 2003). The process of losing parents to HIV/AIDS for the children often includes the pain and the shame of the stigma and the fear that the disease carries in most of our societies (Ljungqvist 2003, Orphans Survey Findings Conference).

Often, children who have lost their parents to AIDS are assumed to be infected with HIV themselves. Once a parent dies, children, particularly girls, may be denied the right to inherit their parents' property as relatives scramble for the belongings of the deceased.

Thus the death of care-givers, coupled with the stigma attached to HIV/AIDS, can put children (particularly girl children) at risk of discrimination, further isolating them from others at a time when they are most vulnerable and need as much care as possible (UNICEF 2004).

Poverty and access to social services

High levels of poverty in Zimbabwe, made worse by the failure of the economy to thrive, have had a significant impact on gender relations and on the vulnerability of girls and women to HIV infection. HIV/AIDS aggravates poverty and poverty aggravates HIV/AIDS. Forty-six per cent of the country's population is classified as very poor and 69 per cent as poor. Unemployment rates are high (50 per cent) and the formal economy has been shrinking. On a per capita basis, GNP (gross national product) has fallen. Against a highly skewed income distribution (among the five worst in the world), the fall in GNP has served to amplify the differences between rich and poor.

Youth and women are disproportionately represented among the poor and unemployed, and their access to opportunity is limited. This background reinforces male dominance and weakens women's ability to negotiate their safety from HIV infection. For girls, sex is a 'currency' through which they are expected to pay for opportunities, favour, and, sometimes, for their survival needs. Issues of safety from HIV infection tend to be secondary. Quite often the exit from poverty 'purchased' through this 'currency' is seen as the most feasible survival strategy.

However, there is an ever-present threat of abandonment. To sustain it, male infidelity has to be tolerated. Within our context today, adult male infidelity is still largely condoned. It would seem this is an abuse of the old understanding of polygamy; nowadays, men do not marry many wives, but instead have several mistresses in a number of places. They may provide for some of these, financially and materially. This has given rise to the phenomenon that is often referred to as the 'small house' – a household made up of younger, economically desperate orphan girls, who see no alternatives to a better life than that offered by a much older man, and who are left vulnerable to HIV infection.

Because of the vulnerability of their situation, orphans and vulnerable children (OVC) are usually the least able to access the resources necessary for basic upkeep. The care of ill parents, who later die of AIDS, usually leaves family resources so depleted that basic rights such as schooling and food can't be afforded. Affected by the structural food deficit that has haunted Zimbabwe over the last couple of years, child-headed households are in a precarious position of trying to balance their need to provide for their basic needs and to be children at the same time (International HIV/ AIDS Alliance 2003).

The economic environment and donor resistance

Having discussed some of the challenges that a girl child has to contend with at an individual level, this section moves on to discuss the challenges at the national level.

The fact that donor aid has been so limited has placed a strain on the locally available resources. According to UNICEF (2004), Zimbabwe receives only a fraction of the HIV/AIDS funding of other countries in the region, despite suffering one of the world's highest rates of HIV/AIDS and a surge in child mortality. UNICEF (2004) also said that in the 2004 to 2005 fiscal year, Zimbabwe received no HIV/AIDS funding support from key global donors in the region. UNICEF goes on to point out that the average annual donor spending per HIV-infected person in Southern Africa from the three agencies stood at $74, but that figure shrunk to just $4 for Zimbabwe. Zimbabwe has been dealt a hard blow in its fight against HIV/AIDS. Other policies such as governments' bans on external support in the form of food aid have wrought havoc in the nation.

Besides the challenges brought on by the absence of funding, Zimbabwe's capacity to respond comprehensively to OVC issues has also been hindered by factors like the hyper-inflationary economic and social conditions, gaps in what has been legislated and what is actually practised in laws and policies protecting OVC, and increasing numbers of OVC and child-headed households but a lack of budgetary allocation for programmes to support them.

Opportunities for the girl child in the face of HIV/AIDS

Despite the challenges Zimbabwe faces in the protection of the girl child from HIV/ AIDS, there still exist some opportunities that can be exploited to improve the life of the girl child:

[W]e must make sure that girls – who run a particular risk of infection – have all the services and self confidence to protect themselves. Across all levels of society we need to see a deep social revolution that transforms relationships between men and women so that women will be able to take greater control of their lives.

Annan (2001)

Clearly, support at the international level for the protection of the girl child is considered a priority. These are opportunities that also need to be explored at both national and community levels.

National level

Zimbabwe has ratified the CRC and CEDAW, which call for the protection of girl children and women in society. It is now a generally accepted reality that the protection of children's rights is closely linked to the realisation and recognition of the rights of women. Jonsson (2003, 25) notes that the CRC and CEDAW are 'complementary and mutually reinforcing'. He goes on to note that girls are particularly at risk of violence, abuse, and HIV infection when gender-based violence is not addressed and inadequate measures are taken to raise women's and girls' overall social status. Therborn (1992) adds that respect for children's rights has always been preceded by an increasing realisation of women's rights. Hence, the protection of the girl child's rights can be strengthened by the realisation of women's rights as well. The fact that Zimbabwe has ratified these two instruments is an opportunity for activists to use them as lobbying tools for government to improve the conditions of the girl child in the face of the HIV/AIDS pandemic. Such conditions may include access to free and compulsory education for the girl child. This means that provisions have to be in place to support children who are care-givers so they can attend school. National priorities therefore have to be revisited, with more budgetary provisions directed towards the protection of the girl child.

Also of importance is Zimbabwe's response to the UN's framework of action. One of the specific goals is to develop national strategies to deal with orphans and other vulnerable children (UNAIDS *et al.* 2004). Zimbabwe is the first in the region to have developed a National Plan of Action for OVC. Given Zimbabwe's commitment to these international protocols, it is important that the government is held accountable to ensure that these are translated into action. Of concern to date is the fact that even though government has made the necessary policy provisions, they are not matched by levels of budgetary allocations. The prioritisation of competing demands, a declining economy, a low revenue base, a rising domestic and foreign service commitment, lack of clear action plans with roles, and targets for operationalising various policies are all contributing to the government's seemingly poor accountability for the rights of the girl child.

Community level

At the community level, HIV/AIDS interventions have tended to focus on communities as targets at which interventions must be aimed. This approach has weakened local creativity and participation. Local participation has tended to be in prescribed roles, mainly those of providing information, material resources, and labour. The spirit of partnership in locally owned intervention has not received adequate attention. Yet, recent experiences with community capacity-building in some districts have revealed the effectiveness of the community in the fight against HIV/AIDS:

> [S]mall, humble but powerful local initiatives in which ordinary people are doing extraordinary things to care for and support children affected by AIDS.

(STRIVE 2003, 8)

Several NGOs are playing strategic roles in the empowerment of children. These include initiatives like those of the Southern African AIDS Trust (SAT), which has set up community-based organisations that are working to alleviate the plight of children and orphans affected/infected by HIV/AIDS, with special focus on the girl child.

Zimbabwe is generally endowed with strong community safety nets that come into play to provide for a family that is in any kind of distress. For instance, a STRIVE project in Gowakowa, Manicaland province, supports orphans and child-headed households by providing them with labour in agricultural fields. Communities also support orphans by providing them with skills in reproductive health issues, a role that would normally be done by an aunt or uncle within the family. The important aspect of the community support for the girl child is that it releases her to attend school and gives her time to be a child, if only for a short while (STRIVE 2005).

Conclusion and recommendations

Support and interventions directed at the girl child should be different and be made to fit into her life (International HIV/AIDS Alliance 2003). UNICEF (2004) notes that within the CRC there is an acknowledgement that even when children face the same challenges as adults they may require different solutions. A rights-based approach should be applied to the promotion of the girl child's well-being. Placing rights at the heart of human development strategies calls for countries to decide which services are essential for vulnerable children, and to be informed by these to create a protective environment (UNICEF 2004).

Some of the solutions to the challenges faced by girls in the face of HIV/AIDS might be as follows.

- Community schools could be created for girls who have to tend to the sick or are household heads (International HIV/AIDS Alliance 2003). The community would own these schools and requirements such as school uniforms would not be as stringent as those of formal schools. Such schools could also be tailored to suit the girls who are disadvantaged in terms of time and attendance.

- Catch-up mechanisms for girls who have not been able to attend school regularly could be explored (International HIV/AIDS Alliance 2003). A local NGO (MAVAMBO) has one such facility and it has proven to be one of the sound models of reintegrating girls who have dropped out of school. Children who have dropped out of school are taught on an individual accelerated basis. The informal learning centre has registered high success rates with graduates from the centre excelling far above those who have been in continuous formal education.

- Discriminatory cultural and traditional practices should be challenged through legislation, matched with the development of enforcement mechanisms to ensure that these are implemented.

- Community mobilisation and participation could be available to support the girl child who has the responsibility of running a home.

- Establishment/strengthening of comprehensive health education and services to reduce the risk of infection should be a priority agenda especially for children who are carers. Coupled with this is the need to increase access to social services.

- Anti-retroviral drugs (ARVs) need to be readily available to families infected by AIDS. This delays death and means the parents will have a longer time in which to be with the children, thereby removing the burden of care, and any responsibilities that would otherwise accrue, from the girl child.

- It is also important that property rights of women and girls are clearly secured. This is also key to addressing the economic hardships they face because of HIV/AIDS.

- It is important that donors invest funds in the girl child. Increased official development assistance is critical for Zimbabwe right now as the country faces a record economic low since independence.

- To strengthen strategies to empower the girl child and make interventions relevant, action-oriented research needs to be undertaken into areas such as: access to ARVs and the related costs and the economic implications for the girl child's family; effective programming for children in a hyper-inflation environment; and gender audits of policies and legislation, with the overall aim of developing transformative actions that will make the girl child's life one based on rights.

The impact of HIV/AIDS on the girl child cannot be addressed at only one level. As nations and communities, there has to be collective responsibility, through which everyone is accountable for the well-being of the girl child. While the immediate and extended families should remain the key source of support for children, it is important that the wider community also shows its responsibility through programmes that are gender sensitive. In a world with AIDS, children must become everybody's priority and responsibility.

This article was originally published in Gender & Development, *volume 14, number 1, March 2006.*

References

Annan, K. (2001) Keynote Address by the Secretary-General of the UN to the Awards Banquet of the Global Health Council Annual Conference, Washington DC.

Bennett-Haigney, L. (2001) 'It Takes a Village to Work for Women's Rights', www.now.org/nnt/spring-2000/profiles.html (last accessed August 2007).

Fredriksson, J. and A. Kanabus (2005) 'AIDS Orphans, the Facts', updated by Jane Penninngton and Annabel Kanabus, May 2005, www.avert.org/aidsorphans.htm (last accessed August 2007).

Guni, F. (2005) 'Death by denial', *Guardian*, London, 30 March 2005.

International HIV/AIDS Alliance (2003) 'Building Blocks: Africa-Wide Briefing Notes', resources for communities working with orphans and vulnerable children, Brighton, UK: International HIV/AIDS Alliance.

Jonsson, U. (2003) 'Human Rights Approach to Development Programming', Nairobi, Kenya: UNICEF, UNAIDS, and USAID.

Ljungqvist, B. (2003) Statement by UNICEF representative, HIV/AIDS Orphans Survey Findings Conference, 8 April 2003, New York.

National Plan of Action (2005) Zimbabwe government document.

Nyamukapa, C., G. Foster, and S. Gregson (2003) 'Orphans' household circumstances and access to education in a maturing epidemic in eastern Zimbabwe', *Journal of Social Development in Africa* 18: 7–32.

STRIVE (2003) 'Mid Term Review Report', May/June 2003, Zimbabwe: Catholic Relief Services.

STRIVE (2005) 'Quarterly Report', April–June 2005, Zimbabwe: Catholic Relief Services.

Therborn, G. (1992) 'Children's Rights in the Constitution of Modern Childhood: A Comparative Study of Western Nations', paper presented at the international conference on Childhood as a Phenomenon: Lessons from an International Project, Bilund, Denmark, 24–26 September 1992.

UNAIDS, UNICEF, and USAID (2004) 'Children on the Brink: A Joint Report of New Orphans Estimates: A Framework for Action', New York: UNICEF.

UNICEF (1998) 'A Study on Children Affected by AIDS in Zimbabwe', www.unicef.org (last accessed August 2007).

UNICEF (2004) *The State of the World's Children*, New York.

Wakhweya, A., M. Kateregga, and C. Konde-Lule (2003) 'Situational Analysis of Orphans and their Households – Caring for the Future Today', Kampala, Uganda: Ministry of Gender and Labour and Social Development.

WHO (1995) 'The Role of the Committee on the Rights of the Child and its Impact on HIV/ AIDS: Problems and Prospects', presentation by the World Health Organization Global Programme on AIDS at AIDS and Child Rights: The Impact on the Asia-Pacific Region, Bangkok, Thailand, 21–26 November 1995.

Zimbabwe Independent (2005) 'More lose homes as Operation Restore Order continues', 24–30 June 2005.

3 'I'm too young to die': HIV, masculinity, danger, and desire in urban South Africa

Shannon Walsh and Claudia Mitchell

'When I passed my grade 8, I started to change, I don't know why. I said that I wanted to be something. So if maybe I kept going out with these guys [pause] about six of them died in the group. So I said, "Not me, I'm not ready to die." So I said, "OK, I must change", so I changed.'

These are the words of KK, an AIDS activist and former gang member in Khayelitsha, South Africa, talking in a videotaped interview that we shot for *Fire and Hope*, a documentary on youth activism. KK reveals on tape that life for him and others like him is 'risky business'. In the video, he pauses as he says this. It is this pause – his unspoken words – that provides a chilling reminder of the danger that is part of an everyday reality for many young men. As we explore here, it is a danger that sits alongside, and intersects with, the risk of HIV infection.

South Africa has one of the largest AIDS epidemics in the world, with prevalence rates resting between 11.4 per cent and 20.1 per cent in the overall population (HSRC 2002; UNAIDS 2002). Infection rates in young people continue to increase. There is now a clear recognition of some of the factors that place girls and young women at greater risk of infection than young men. These range from greater biological vulnerability to greater social vulnerability. Social factors in vulnerability include sex undertaken for material gain, sexual relationships between younger women and older men, and violence against women. Yet, in our ongoing action-oriented and participatory research with young men and women around HIV prevention, we have been struck by other aspects of gender identity and gender relations. These include the commonplace discussion of gangs and violence among young urban males, and the effect of that violence on their perception of risk, sexuality, and death. Robert Morrell writes, 'In South Africa, violent masculinities have been more in evidence and the colonial past longer and more oppressive than in most countries around the world' (Morrell 2005, 273). This history is not one that will be easily changed, even with the imperative of the AIDS crisis.

Researchers have begun to look at gender relations in the context of township violence, as factors in HIV risk (Selikow *et al.* 2002). As the 2001 Medical Research Council report warned gravely, 80 per cent of today's 15-year-old South African boys are likely to die before the age of 60 (MRC 2001). In this context, it is essential to develop systems to prevent HIV among young people, including providing education, and providing services to support those who have contracted the virus. At the same time, the process of creating successful prevention campaigns has been daunting and ineffective, causing young people increasingly to exclaim their sense of being 'sick of AIDS' education (Mitchell and Smith 2003).

In this article, we are interested in the intersections between violence, gangsterism,[1] and perceived HIV risk, in relation to the lives of boys and young men. Glaser writes, 'Juvenile criminality and youth gangs emerged almost organically out of the social and economic dead ends that township youths faced throughout the 1930s, 1940s, and 1950s' (2000, 41). In the context of family instability, unemployment, overcrowding of family homes, inadequate schooling, poverty and little hope for a future with decent economic prospects, 'gang life seemed attractive; it offered companionship, a sense of belonging, and a possible means of income' (*ibid.*).

Gangs, violence, and male identity in South Africa's urban areas

Gangsterism is an acknowledged problem in South Africa, with the coloured[2] communities in the Western Cape some of the most inundated by gang-related activity and violence (Glaser 2000; Leggett 2004). Ted Leggett, of the Institute for Security Studies, reminds us that 'official figures suggest that coloured people are twice as likely as any other ethnic group to be murdered, and twice as likely to be incarcerated' (Leggett 2004, 21). People in the coloured population are far more likely to be killed or be victims of violent crime than any other group in South Africa (Leggett 2004). According to Leggett, the reasons for the high levels of violent crime and incarceration include: pressured idleness in relation to unemployment; claustrophobia in relation to densely populated living quarters; substance abuse; and gangsterism. Leggett sees a direct link between the overcrowded housing situation and tightly populated living quarters in coloured communities, and the fact that many youths end up out on the streets, creating new 'homes' and families on the block. Those relationship dynamics quickly form into street-level gangs.

In his book *Street Gangs throughout the World*, Herbert C. Covey argues that street gangs are becoming an increasingly important area of cultural study (Covey 2003). The number of impoverished street children in the world with few socio-economic options in life is increasing, while, at the same time, street gangs can be seen to represent opportunities for young men to gain social status, a sense of security and community, and the possibility of potential economic gain. In South Africa, with the growing number of AIDS orphans, this situation is likely to get worse.

A substantial amount of scholarly work has been done on gang activity in South Africa (Glaser 2000; Houston and Prinsloo 1998; Pinnock and Douglas-Hamilton 1997, 1998). Gangs have been present in South Africa at least as far back as the turn of the twentieth century (Covey 2003; Kynoch 1999). There are varying theories about the reasons behind substantial gang activity in South Africa, which we cannot give justice to in this chapter, but a surface reading of motivations for gangsterism is enlightening. Covey (2003), citing Pinnock (1995), notes the ways in which gangsterism in the Cape Flats is a response to the forced removals under apartheid that left people displaced and without community cohesion. In this theory, youth drifted towards gangs and street-level communities in response to what they were lacking in terms of community, protection, leadership, and social control. Glaser takes the opposing view, claiming that forced removals were not the primary cause of the gang activity, but rather high levels of community and neighbourhood loyalty drove youth to join street gangs (2000). Steinberg (2004) in his analysis of the 26s and 28s gangs speaks as well of an enforced insularity once communities had been removed from their previous lives closer to the centre of Cape Town. Whatever the actual motivating factors, scholars agree that gangs are a significant aspect of young male lives in the townships of South Africa.

Published autobiographies show us that the high risks associated with gang life and life on the streets are not new. Examples are William Modisane's account of growing up in Sophiatown in the late 1920s and early 1930s, or Rrekgetsi Chimeloane's narrative of 1960s boyhood in Diepkloof in Soweto (Chimeloane 2005; Modisane 2005). Modisane notes that death was just part of the everyday: 'We were part of the riot programme, stoning the police and being shot at, and hit, like everyone else. I learned early in life to play games with death, to realise its physical presence in my life, to establish rapport with it. The children of Sophiatown died in the streets, being run over by the Putco buses and the speeding taxis, and were shot during riots' (136). A particularly dramatic account can be seen in Jonny Steinberg's book *The Number*, a biography of Magadien Wentzel, a coloured prisoner of Polsmoor Prison, with a lifelong career in the 28s (a well-known South African gang). Speaking of the forced relocation of people from District Six to the Cape Flats,[3] Steinberg describes the situation that created gang territories and identity:

> *The new neighbourhoods of the Cape Flats were to become deeply insular. Each block came to constitute a territory, its defenders possessive of insiders, aggressive to outsiders ...The ghettos of the Flats were divided into hundreds of microturfs, each given life by a micro-identity ...It extended to who did*

business with whom, how one earned a living, and, perhaps most important of all, the politics of street gangs, which drew entire communities into their wars.

Steinberg (2004, 114)

Linking gangsterism and violence to HIV/AIDS responses

We highlight these accounts both to provide historical context for violence and gangs, and to add a new part to the equation. What does it mean to construct a 'healthy sexuality', and to protect yourself from HIV infection, illness, and death, when you are a witness, perpetrator, or victim of violent crime? What are boys' perceptions of risk in a context where death and danger haunt each of their movements? How do constructions of masculine identity that include sexual domination of women inhibit boys from seeing that they can still feel masculine while having safe sex? Attention has been paid to how male violence against women and girls increases the vulnerability of girls to HIV. But, based on our findings in contexts such as Atlantis and Khayelitsha, we consider it is time for a more nuanced investigation into gender violence. In particular, how do economic poverty, widespread violence, and gang-related activity create the dominant ideas about what it means to be a man in locations such as these? This creates an extremely risky environment for young people as regards the possibility of HIV infection.

The challenge for educators and researchers is to understand the conflicts and contradictions in 'coming of age' sexually, when young people are starkly aware of extreme violence and the daily possibility of death. Along with others (Bhana 2005; Pattman 2002), we would like to argue that more attention needs to be given to the realities of young people's lives in order to create strategies that actually respond to their needs.

Voices from the project

To that end, in the sections that follow, we discuss the experience of several young men. Each participated in an arts-based AIDS-prevention project, in which they talked and wrote on the topic of 'in my neighbourhood'. These narratives eventually became part of a small published volume entitled *In My Life: Youth Stories and Poems about HIV and AIDS*. In addition, a set of writings and drawings was produced locally, called *Voices from Atlantis: Young People Write and Illustrate the Impact of HIV/AIDS on their Lives*.[4] It was in this context as researchers working within the project that we began to learn something of the everyday stories of masculinities situated within the histories of these particular communities, which, while less than a 45-minute drive away from each other on the Cape peninsula, represent very different realities.

Gangsterism and desire

Atlantis sits about 60km up the coast from Cape Town. Located among the rolling sand dunes of the outer edges of the Cape, Atlantis is a factory town. It has a population of almost 50,000 coloured people, who relocated there during the years of apartheid. They came mainly from areas such as District Six. Atlantis is marked by high levels of unemployment, and many residents make the daily journey into Paarl or Cape Town in search of work. The physical infrastructure of Atlantis is not as poor as the 'townships' that had indigenous African populations during apartheid. There are few shacks or shanties, yet people live in close quarters, which are often overpopulated. Atlantis lies on the outskirts of the gang-ridden area of the Cape Flats, and, like much of the Western Cape, is a hotspot of gang activity (Pinnock 1987). In working with young men in this context, it is no surprise that gangsterism as a topic provides real and tangible examples of the ways in which boys grow to think of themselves as male, and how they understand their own vulnerabilities. Indeed, when asked during an HIV-prevention workshop to write a short piece on the topic of 'something that happened in my neighbourhood', 11 out of 13 young people at a local secondary school in Atlantis wrote about witnessing a murder or violent crime. As 16-year-old Clinton writes:

> *In some neighbourhoods not much strange things happen*
>
> *but on one specific day*
>
> *something you have nightmares about happens*
>
> *and you are involved*
>
> *and almost pay with your life.*
>
> *You ask yourself 'where is the love?'*
>
> *and some people just tell you*
>
> *shut up*
>
> *shut up*
>
> *shut up*

Clinton, aged 16, 'In my neighbourhood', excerpt from *Voices from Atlantis*, p. 5

Clinton has a very real sense that his life was in danger at the time he describes here. Understanding how real this sense of death and dying is for young men is critical to unpacking the potential of HIV-prevention campaigns, especially in terms of their ability to make positive life choices and steer clear of fatally dangerous behaviour. If young men are living in an environment of extreme violence, where life is seen as insignificant or highly risky, the ability and desire to protect themselves from AIDS may well seem of minor importance. Not only that, but love, equated with sex, itself may be used as an escape from violent surroundings. As Clinton laments, 'where is the love?'. Selikow *et al.* (2002) note in their analysis of HIV/AIDS and township youth culture in Alexandra that many young people feel that since 'one's time to die is predetermined, it is not necessary to protect oneself against the possibility of AIDS' (25). They also suggest that the dangers and perils of daily township life may often seem more tangible than dangers associated with AIDS (Selikow *et al.* 2002). How can young men be encouraged towards health-enabling strategies geared towards taking care of themselves and their future, if that future is so uncertain?

The challenge to change

Khayelitsha is a densely populated informal urban township, sprawling with shacks and dirt roads. With almost 500,000 people living in close quarters, Khayelitsha is one of South Africa's largest townships. It is no wonder that young men turn to gangsterism, given the contexts of poverty, poor schooling, racism, overcrowding, violence, and bleak future prospects. In our sessions, young people discussed and wrote a great deal about what life was like, and their sadness, joy, and fear.

Nosbusiso, a 17-year-old girl, wrote a story that reflects many of the intersecting, and sometimes opposing, ideas of masculinity in the context of gang violence:

It happened in my Neighbourhood ...

It was 6:30pm, just when the Bold and Beautiful ended. The boy's mother asked him if he would go and buy sugar and potatoes and a packet of tea bags. He said, 'Yes I can, right after Jam Alley.'

His mother said, 'That's okay, I will only cook at 7 o'clock anyway.'

'Thanks Mom', he said.

'What for?', his mother asked.

'Just about everything, but mostly for not yelling at me when I said I will go after Jam Alley.'

Then she said, 'You are welcome.' She gave him a hug.

When Jam Alley ended, he went out. As he went down the passage a drunk old man said to him, 'You better watch yourself son, there is a lot of violence outside there.'

When he stepped on the pavement there were thugs shooting at one another, and a shot hit him behind his neck. He fell on the road and a motor car hit him. When another one hit him, this time it was a taxi. He went up into the sky. When he was just about fallen down another one hit him again. His mother heard the shots. She came running. She said, 'Please God, don't let it be my son.'

When she saw it was her son she said, 'Ooh my God! Not my baby. Please it can't be.'

Nosbusiso, excerpt from *In My Life*, p. 22

Nosbusiso's story presents a kind and sensitive boy who is a victim of gang violence. The sense that 'outside' is a dangerous place comes through clearly in her story. This life of fear and danger is one that 17-year-old Thembi, who also participated in the session, could expect to experience in Khayelitsha. Thembi was a part of a gang himself in his early teens, but he left the gang when he realised that his life was in danger. He began working as a peer educator on HIV prevention and treatment, and had become recognised in the community as someone knowledgeable about HIV and AIDS. Interestingly, gang members who still remembered him from the old days began to consult Thembi for advice. Most of the gang members are out of school, and comprise one of the hardest groups to reach with prevention programmes and education. Thembi talked about how gang members would question him on condoms, myths they had heard about AIDS, and other sex-related questions. At the same time, during our interviews, Thembi's ideas about what it means to be a man in this community surfaced:

> Thembi: 'Have the discussion about condoms outside [the bedroom] ...whereby she won't get hurt, you see.'
>
> Interviewer: 'Because you mean when you are in the bedroom it is more dangerous? To say, "use a condom" at that moment?'
>
> Thembi: 'Let's say I say, "OK, it's been a year now, and we never have had sex, but today is a good day" ...so they go after school. And the girl then, she will refuse. And I will say, "No, you are mad! You can't [refuse], you see." What we are saying, what boys are saying is, "When I took you home to here, what was going on in your mind at that time? Did you think I would just go with you and bring you here?" [lots of laughing and talking in room]

At the time of writing, we understand that Thembi has recently rejoined the gangs he fought so hard to separate himself from. This reminds us that issues of poverty and violence are realities in the townships that are not going to change overnight, especially when young people have few other options.

Scholars agree that the assertion and confirmation of dominant ideas about being a man are an important part of gangsterism. Gang members were admired for fighting skill, success with women, and criminal daring, which often included rape (Glaser 2000). Being part of a youth gang was understood as a strong expression of young urban masculinity (*ibid.*). Women are, in this context, most often 'viewed as property of the gang, and [are] expected to be loyal to their gang boyfriends' (Covey 2003, 178). Most of the boys in our study were not (or did not admit to being) involved in gangs themselves. They were oppressed by the violence they encountered in their environment, yet were influenced by the particular understandings of masculine identity that gang culture perpetuates. This understanding includes sexual violence aimed towards women.

This kind of reality has serious implications for policy makers on HIV/AIDS. Unfortunately men in South Africa are still not generally supportive of organisations or campaigns that 'identify men's responsibility for violence and inequality and work towards gender justice' (Morrell 2005, 279). As we saw in the case of Thembi, even while he was interested in changing the situation around HIV and AIDS, he still understood male/female relationships in terms of the potential for violence, and men's right to exert that violence over women.

Various researchers have aptly pointed out that oversimplifying culturally dominant notions of what it means to be a man as fundamentally oppressive, violent, and subjugating to women is not helpful: it limits our ability to understand the existence of other ideas that co-exist with the dominant idea (Pattman 2002; Thorpe 2002). At the same time, it is necessary to look at the ways in which boys are recreating these realities and how they may also be contesting them. Certainly, in the mixed discussions with our youth groups, there were moments when boys showed their vulnerability and uncertainties around sex. Shaheen, slightly younger than Clinton and Thembi, expressed his concern about condom use: 'It seems to the girl like I'm trying to pressure her if I bring out a condom.'

Shaheen's perspective, in contrast to some of the more dominant masculinities we observed, was concerned with even *appearing* to pressure a girl to have sex. Shaheen brought forth the rarely discussed power dynamics young men might be subject to around negotiating condom use. Shaheen reminds us about the difficulties young men have in revealing uncertainty and vulnerability around sexuality. Spaces must be created for young men to investigate their own vulnerabilities and fears around sexual relationships.

Context is critical

Catherine Campbell argues that 'people are most likely to undergo health-enhancing behaviour change if they live in communities that offer high levels of participation in local networks and organisations, which are associated with increased levels of trust, reciprocal help and support, and a positive local community identity' (2003, 9). Members of the community need to feel that their 'views are respected and valued' (51), and that 'they have channels to participate in making decisions in the context of family, school and neighbourhood' (*ibid.*).

In the cases we are discussing here, we would argue that this process is constrained by an environment overrun with gangs and violence, as well as by dominant views of masculine identity that condone violence against women, and sexism. At the same time, for some youth, gangs might be the only spaces in which young men, who are otherwise oppressed by the dominant society on various fronts, feel they have the ability to make important decisions that are respected and valued.

Norman, a 15-year-old resident of Atlantis, wrote in his *Voices from Atlantis* story that his context has 'never been the same again' since he became aware of a woman's murder:

There are trees

Just down the road.

A woman was killed there The guy who killed her

Cut off the side of her face

Her cheek

Since then,

Our peaceful,

Quiet, neighbourhood

Has never been the same again.

Norman, excerpt from *Voices from Atlantis*, p. 3

This young author sees the gendered nature of a man killing a woman. At the same time, he records the shift in the way he saw his neighbourhood, which turned, for him, into a place in which he doesn't feel safe. His story reminds us how violence affects the ways in which individuals see their home communities, turning them from safe and positive places into places of risk and danger. If we are convinced that trust and positive relationships within the community are important for adequate and effective HIV prevention, then the context of circular violence, gender inequality, and poverty must be addressed as part of AIDS campaigns.

Implications, recommendations, and conclusions

Gang and street-level violence within communities, as well as high levels of sexual violence among young people, must be seriously considered as situational elements affecting the ways boys construct their identities and HIV vulnerability. Given the context in which boys find themselves, we feel it is necessary to outline some strategies to integrate into work on sexuality and HIV prevention with youth.

First, appraisals of the lived experience of boys and young men in relation to violence should be incorporated into all programme planning. It is critical to step beyond only seeing boys as perpetrators of sexual violence and gang violence, to listen closely to their stories and experience as a way to begin to unpack their own constructed masculine identities, which value violence, dominance, and sexual persuasion and ownership of girls. Young men should be included in gender analysis of the contexts in which HIV service-providers work. They need to be given conceptual tools and methods that help them understand the social conditioning that leads them to think that being a man involves risk, danger, and violence. They also need to be nurtured in their own self-esteem to combat the hopelessness, bleak futures, and sense that 'it doesn't matter anyway, because I will die soon'. Boys must be supported in creating positive self-images and positive strategies for their own futures, and the idea that there are different and more positive ways to think about being a man should be promoted.

At the same time, we need to develop prevention strategies that understand the realities of the violence, hopelessness, and recklessness that exist for boys in South Africa today. While changing these realities must be a top priority, we must also develop ways to integrate condom use, for example, into relationships that continue to exist in hegemonic forms (for example strategies that associate condom use with strength, conviction, and responsibility for 'taking care of the girls'). Too much is at stake to have HIV prevention resting solely on the entire transformation of social realities.

In looking at boys' and young men's sexual and masculine identities, we must bear in mind their relationships to their broader context and community. Violence and gangsterism affect their understanding of risk, their concept of how long they will live, their sense of self-worth, and their sense of the impact of risky behaviour on their lives. All these issues should be investigated more thoroughly. We follow Selikow *et al.* in their claim that 'it will be difficult to encourage new forms of culture until current economic realities are challenged', yet also their view that 'safer sexual practices can be encouraged while current cultural practices prevail' (2002, 30). At the same time, without looking more deeply at how some of the factors we have noted above affect young masculine identities, we will only have a partial picture of boys' lives and their abilities to be agents in a 'health-enabling community'.

This article was originally published in Gender & Development, *volume 14, number 1, March 2006.*

References

Bhana, D. (2005) 'Violence and the gendered negotiation of masculinity among young black school boys in South Africa', in L. Ouzgane and R. Morrell (eds.) *African Masculinities: Men in Africa from the Late Nineteenth Century to the Present,* New York: Palgrave MacMillan, pp. 205–20.

Campbell, C. (2003) *'Letting Them Die': Why HIV/AIDS Prevention Programmes Fail,* Bloomington, IN: Indiana University Press.

Chimeloane, R. (2005) 'Who's laetie are you?', in A. Hadland (ed.) *Childhood: South Africans Recall Their Past,* Johannesburg: Penguin.

Covey, H. C. (2003) *Street Gangs throughout the World,* Springfield, IL: Charles C. Thomas Publishers, Ltd.

Glaser, C. (2000) Bo Tsotsi: *The Youth Gangs of Soweto 1935 –1976,* Oxford: James Currey.

Houston, J. and J. Prinsloo (1998) 'Prison gangs in South Africa: a comparative analysis', *Journal of Gang Research* 5(3).

HSRC (2002) *Nelson Mandela/HSRC Study of HIV/AIDS: South African National HIV Prevalence, Behavioural Risks and Mass Media*, Cape Town: Human Science Research Council Publishers.

HSRC (2004) *The National Household HIV Prevalence and Risk Survey of South African Children*, Cape Town: Human Science Research Council Publishers.

Kynoch, G. (1999) 'From the Ninevites to the Hard Livings gang: township gangsters and urban violence in twentieth-century South Africa', *African Studies* 58(1): 55–85.

Leggett, T. (2004) 'Still marginal: crime in the coloured community', *SA Crime Quarterly* 7: 21–6.

Mitchell, C. and A. Smith (2003) 'Sick of AIDS: literacy and the meaning of life for South African youth', *Culture, Health & Sexuality* 5(6): 513–22.

Modisane, W. B. (2005) 'Blame me on history', in A. Hadland (ed.) *Childhood: South Africans Recall Their Past*, Johannesburg: Penguin, pp. 135–44.

Morrell, R. (2001) *Changing Men in Southern Africa*, Pietermaritzburg and London: University of Natal Press and Zed Books Ltd.

Morrell, R. (2005) 'Men, movements, and gender transformations in South Africa', in L. Ouzgane and R. Morrell (eds.) *African Masculinities: Men in Africa from the Late Nineteenth Century to the Present*, New York: Palgrave MacMillan, pp. 271–88.

MRC (2001) *The Impact of HIV/AIDS on Adult Mortality in South Africa*, Tygerberg: Medical Research Council.

Pattman, R. (2002) 'Men make a difference: the construction of gendered student identities at the University of Botswana', *Agenda* 53: 33–42.

Pinnock, D. (1987) 'Stone's boys and the making of a Cape Flats mafia', in B. Bozzoli (ed.) *Class, Community and Conflict*, Johannesburg: Ravan Press.

Pinnock, D. (1995) 'Suffer the little children', *Democracy in Action*, 8–9.

Pinnock, D. and M. Douglas-Hamilton (1997) *Gangs, Rituals and Rites of Passage*, Cape Town: African Sun Press with the Institute of Criminology, University of Cape Town.

Pinnock, D. and M. Douglas-Hamilton (1998) 'Rituals, rights, and tradition: rethinking youth programs in South Africa', in K. Hazlehurst and C. Hazlehurst (eds.) *Gangs and Youth Subcultures: International Explorations*, New Brunswick, NJ: Transaction.

Schuster, A. (ed.) (2003) *In My Life: Youth Stories and Poems about HIV and AIDS*, Cape Town: Center for the Book.

Selikow, T., B. Zulu, and E. Cedras (2002) 'The Ingagara, the regte and the cherry: HIV/ AIDS and youth culture in contemporary urban townships', *Agenda* 53: 22–32.

Steinberg, J. (2004) *The Number: One Man's Search for Identity in the Cape Underworld and Prison Gangs*, Johannesburg and Cape Town: Jonathan Ball Publishers.

Thorpe, M. (2002) 'Masculinity in an HIV intervention', *Agenda* 53: 61–8.

UNAIDS (2002) *South Africa*, Epidemiological Fact Sheets on HIV/ AIDS and Sexually Transmitted Infections, Geneva: UNAIDS, WHO Working Group on Global HIV/ AIDS.

Notes

1 'Gangsterism' is a term popularly used in South Africa to indicate the social phenomenon of violent gangs.

2 The term 'coloured' was established by the apartheid regime to denote South Africans who were the progeny of racially mixed couples. Given the dominant discourse in relation to white supremacy, these people were seen to represent the visible evidence of miscegenation that was strenuously legislated against at the time. The term reflects the racist history of apartheid: so-called coloured people suffered discrimination from both sides of the racial divide in their being neither black nor white. These people were treated appallingly, as outcasts. In response to this, they established close-knit communities, developed a patois of their own out of their predominantly Afrikaans linguistic heritage, and formed many other cultural bonds. Because they are mostly of a lighter skin colour than black South Africans, those who were of Malay descent became caught up in this taxonomy as well. Therefore it is important to regard coloured people as a social/cultural group, which is why we have chosen to use this term here, even though such terms are falling into disuse.

3 District Six was a vibrant mixed neighbourhood in Cape Town, where people of all races had lived in harmony from the late 1800s. In 1966, it was declared a white area by the apartheid government and over the next 15 years 60,000 people were forcibly moved to the Cape Flats – an inhospitable area with almost no amenities at all.

4 *Voices from Atlantis* emerged from workshops conducted and developed by youth HIV activists in Atlantis including Chinomy Jacobs, Mathew Johannes, Kaylene Schroeder, and Danlia Weiner as part of Master's research by Shannon Walsh. The project was made possible through the support of CBIE/CIDA. *In My Life: Youth Stories and Poems about HIV and AIDS* was published by the Center for the Book and came out of an arts-based HIV-prevention project aimed at youth in Cape Town and led by Claudia Mitchell. We acknowledge the support of CIDA/CSIH/ICAD's Small Grants Fund as well as the Social Sciences and Humanities Research Council.

4 A gendered response to HIV/AIDS in South Asia and the Pacific: insights from the pandemic in Africa

Madhu Bala Nath

Currently, one in every five people newly infected with HIV worldwide lives in the Asia and Pacific region. According to the 2004 UNAIDS report on HIV, in all, over 8 million people were living with the virus in the region at the end of 2003 as compared to 42 million across the globe. More than a quarter – 2.6 million – are young people aged between 15 and 24. The year 2003 also saw half a million deaths due to AIDS in the Asia and Pacific region, as against 3 million deaths globally. An addition of 1 million new infections happened in Asia in 2003, compared to 5 million worldwide (all statistics from UNAIDS 2004).

These figures show that the epidemic in the Asia and Pacific region has not reached the level seen in sub-Saharan Africa, where the total number of people living with HIV/AIDS today stands at 29 million (*ibid.*). Yet the current trends indicate that the Asia and Pacific region could replace sub-Saharan Africa as the centre of the global HIV/AIDS epidemic over the next decade, in terms of the absolute number of people affected. In 2010, the number of new HIV infections in Asia and the Pacific is predicted to be 18.5 million, as compared to 21 million new infections in sub-Saharan Africa in the same year (Stover *et al.* 2002). In just two countries of this region, China and India, an estimated 5 million people are already living with HIV/AIDS (*ibid.*). Official estimates predict a ten-fold increase in people living with HIV/AIDS in China by 2010.

Many locations within Asia already have HIV prevalence rates as high as the African countries. For example, prevalence rates among men who have sex with men in several Malaysian states are around 10 per cent. Similarly, in India, red-light areas in Mumbai and Chennai are recording HIV prevalence rates of 55 per cent. In China's Yunan province, and in Myitkyina province in Burma, rates of up to 40 per cent have been detected. These high figures contrast with the national prevalence rates for India and China, which are 0.8 per cent and 0.4 per cent respectively. In Burma, the national prevalence is estimated at 1 per cent, yet prevalence rates among injecting drug users (IDUs) and sex workers are as high as 60 per cent and 40 per cent respectively (Monitoring the AIDS Pandemic 2001, 2).

However, prevalence rates are inadequate as warning systems in the Asia and Pacific region. In view of the region's large population base, even a low prevalence rate shows that huge numbers of people are infected with HIV. As an example, a rise of just 0.1 per cent in India's national HIV prevalence rate would increase the national total of Indian adults living with HIV by half a million.

The factors that make Asia and the Pacific vulnerable

There are a number of factors of concern that are making the Asia and Pacific region vulnerable to HIV/AIDS. Some of these are features of most societies in the region; others are more location-specific. In this section, I discuss each of these in turn.

Unequal gender relations

Some people consider HIV/AIDS to be confined to particular sub-sections of Asian and Pacific society – sex workers, drug users, migrant workers, men who have sex with men. There is also a belief that sex with multiple partners is not common in Asian and Pacific societies. There is a widespread assumption that Asian and Pacific societies will be safe from the worst of the global HIV/AIDS epidemic because – to paraphrase the words that I have often heard from supposedly educated and informed people – 'our culture will save us'.

Yet this is simply not the case. The empirical evidence from the region points to the contrary. The epidemic in Asia and the Pacific is inextricably linked to the power relations between, and among, men and women. Just as in Africa, social stereotypes of male sexual behaviour encourage men to exhibit their 'masculinity' through displays of sexual prowess. These include having multiple sex partners. Many Asian and Pacific men have sexual relations with multiple partners. Men may also display masculinity by indulging in alcohol and other substances. This state of affairs has negative repercussions for women, who have to face unsafe sex and violence. Young women and girls are particularly susceptible.

A study in Thailand has found that 17 per cent of men aged 17 to 45 were part of 'bridging populations' – that is, they had sex with both sex workers and regular partners and spouses, and served as a bridge allowing the virus to cross into different sections of society (National AIDS Control Organization, Ministry of Health and Family Welfare, Government of India 2001). In Bangladesh, a higher proportion of men buy sex than anywhere else in the region, and female sex workers in Bangladesh report the lowest condom use in the region. It is worth noting here that over 80 per cent of women in Asia who have been infected had not placed themselves at risk in similar ways. Instead, they appear to have been infected in what they regarded as monogamous relationships with their husbands and boyfriends.

In many Asian and Pacific societies, just as in African societies, the promotion of safe sexual practices is made more difficult by cultures of silence that surround sex and sexuality. Social expectations of 'good women' (who are contrasted with the 'bad women', with whom men have illicit, often paid, sexual relations) require that they remain ignorant about their sexuality, are passive and subservient to men, and give up autonomous control over their bodies. Lack of economic independence and low social status restricts women's ability to discuss fidelity and insist on condom use. A study of low-income women in long-term relationships in Mumbai, India illustrates how economic dependency has a negative effect on women's ability to control their bodies. In addition to believing that they held too little economic leverage to alter their husbands' behaviour, the women believed that the economic disadvantages of leaving even abusive relationships far outweighed the health risks of staying in those relationships (Shalini 2000). One study in Viet Nam found that only 35 per cent of the women felt able to refuse sex to their husbands (UNIFEM 2002).

Even if safe sex is an option within a particular relationship, in practice this means a woman must give up hope of bearing children. This would be a source of sadness for many women, regardless of social pressures to have children, but it is all the more difficult for women who are expected by family and community to bear children as the ultimate sign of womanhood, of feminine ideals, and of wifely duty.

Low levels of sexual and reproductive health

Another factor is that sexual and reproductive health services are not adequate to prevent infections or support those already infected. The statistics from South Asia are alarming. The prevalence of HIV in sexually transmitted disease (STD) clinic attendees in Pune in India was 43 per cent (UNAIDS 2004). Only 12 per cent of women in Bihar and Gujarat (two states in India) know that condoms can prevent HIV/AIDS (National AIDS Control Organization, Ministry of Health and Family Welfare, Government of India 2001).

As noted above, several countries in the region are harbouring serious local epidemics, where prevalence rates are many times higher than the national prevalence rates. These are locations where, in addition to underlying gender inequality, there are also one or more factors that place populations particularly at risk.

Women's increasing dependence on men in higher-income households

There have been increases in disposable incomes within some sections of Asian societies, and this is associated with the growth of inequality, both between and within households. If household incomes go up as a result of men being able to earn more than previously, gender inequality within the household can worsen, in the sense that male breadwinners may decide that women should no longer engage in income-generating activities themselves, but should remain within the home as housewives. This leads to the total economic dependency of wives on their husbands, and weakens wives' bargaining power when decisions have to be made. Women who cannot make decisions about when and how to have sex cannot protect themselves from HIV/AIDS.

In other households, women have lost their outside employment due to the tumbling of the Asian tigers[1] a few years ago. The Asian financial crisis has created a scale of deprivation in the region that is perhaps unprecedented, and is essentially tilted against women. Korea saw a tripling of unemployment between 1997 and 1998. In Thailand, 1.2 million workers lost their jobs (more than 50 per cent of whom were women). Indonesia slashed its wages by 34 per cent in real terms in the formal urban sector, and by 40 per cent in agriculture. Currency devaluation has resulted in wages losing value, and government cuts in social spending have created further strain on the household. The government of Thailand cut its budget for HIV-related work by 25 per cent in 1998, and in Indonesia the nominal health budget for 1998 was cut by 4 per cent from its 1997 level. In real terms, the cut was much higher owing to the rising inflation (57.6 per cent) in 1998 (ESCAP 2002a). This situation has made both women and men more vulnerable to the epidemic in the region.

Increased migration and mobility

A factor that makes Asia particularly vulnerable to HIV/AIDS is that, over the last decade, the region has witnessed fast economic development. This has led to an expansion of transport systems, resulting in infrastructure that is comparatively well-developed in areas where economic development and employment opportunities are limited. This encourages people to migrate for work, and results in a highly mobile population.

Impoverishment and involvement in the sex industry

In households in which economic change has led to further impoverishment, sex work may be the last resort. Sex workers are often young, generally poor, have had no education, and tend to come from rural and resource-poor settings. Many depend on sex work to support their parents and families. As sex work is illegal in the region, sex workers live and work at the discretion of enforcement agencies. Harassment and discrimination leave sex workers particularly vulnerable to HIV/AIDS.

The tumbling of the Asian tigers has occurred at the same time as huge increases in HIV prevalence rates among sex workers in the region. The prevalence rate among sex workers in the Guangxi province of China rose from 0 per cent in 1996 to 10 per cent in 2000. Similarly the prevalence rates among brothel-based sex workers in Mumbai in India skyrocketed, from just 1 per cent to 51 per cent between 1987 and 1998. In Viet Nam's main cities of Hanoi and Ho Chi Minh, HIV prevalence rates among sex workers rose sharply in the late 1990s from 0 per cent in 1994 to as high as 25 per cent in 2000. The rates in parts of Burma jumped from 4.3 to 18 per cent in three years. As suggested earlier, a rise in the HIV/AIDS prevalence rate among sex workers signals a likely increase in HIV among the 'faithful' wives of the clients of sex workers.

Drug production and use

Another factor that makes the Asia and Pacific region vulnerable to a huge increase in HIV infection is that two of the major production sites for illegal drugs are located here. This has serious implications for the spread of HIV. The most conservative estimate of HIV prevalence among injecting drug users in the Asia and Pacific region numbers in millions. Data also show that HIV prevalence among injecting drug users could be as high as 54 per cent in pockets of Thailand, 85.7 per cent in pockets of China, 80 per cent in pockets of India, and 89 per cent in pockets of Viet Nam (Sarkar 2003).

Sharing needles and syringes is not the only risk. Young (generally male) injectors are also sexually active, often with multiple partners, and often do not practise safe sex. In Pakistan, a behavioural survey in Quetta recorded that over half of injecting drug users visited sex workers, and very few had ever used a condom (UNAIDS 2004). Evidence from Jakarta shows that many injecting drug users have casual sex with multiple partners, usually without using a condom. In Da Nang in Viet Nam, over 20 per cent of injecting drug users had paid for sex in the previous year. In Hanoi, the figure was 25 per cent, and most of them had not used a condom (Monitoring the AIDS Pandemic 2001). Similarly, between 50 per cent and 75 per cent of male injecting drug users in Bangladesh paid for sex with women, and nearly 10 per cent paid for sex with other men. The impact of this on non-paid sex partners is dramatic. Approximately 45 per cent of the wives of injecting drug users in Manipur in India were found to be HIV-positive (ESCAP/UNDCP/UNAIDS 2001).

The impact of HIV/AIDS on African countries: how can we avoid this in Asia?

In September 2000, the heads of state of a number of African countries declared HIV/AIDS a national disaster at the African Summit on HIV/AIDS held in Addis Ababa, Ethiopia. A declaration of a national disaster signifies recognition of the inability of systems of governance to respond to a challenge. Two decades of responding to the challenge of HIV has shown us the direct link between governance and HIV. In part, it was good governance that halted, or plateaued, the epidemic in countries like

Thailand, Uganda, Senegal, Brazil, Australia, the USA, and the countries of Europe. Access to treatment and access to prevention technology were facilitated by these states in response to demands from citizens.

In the countries of sub-Saharan Africa where the pandemic gained a hold, there is both empirical and anecdotal evidence to show that HIV/AIDS has undone development gains, upset development goals, and skewed development targets. Child mortality rates have increased by 30 per cent in some countries because of perinatal transmission; infant mortality is projected to be 60 per cent higher than it would have been without HIV/AIDS. In Botswana, as early as 1997, life expectancy had fallen to 52 years (it was 65 years until 1996). The UNDP Human Poverty Index (with components of longevity, deprivation of knowledge, and deprivation of living standards) and the Human Development Index (with components of life expectancy, literacy, and per capita income) are very sensitive to the impact of HIV/AIDS (UNDP 1996). UNDP-supported studies indicate that many countries have lost years of Table progress.[2]

Table: Loss of progress (over 30 years) against three indicators of human development

Country	Loss of progress in number of years
Zambia	10
Tanzania	8
Rwanda	7
Central African Republic	6
Burundi, Kenya, Malawi, Uganda	3-5

Source: *Human Development Report*, 1997, UNDP

At a national level, the HIV epidemic in South Asia could drain national and human resources, right down to the community and household level. In countries in which the HIV epidemic is mature or maturing, the financial and material burden of care tends to shift away from overburdened hospitals towards families. As more and more people living with HIV move into the advanced phase of the disease, in which they contract AIDS-related illnesses, recurrent and protracted bouts of illness place an additional burden on already poor households. As in Africa, women in countries in Asia and the Pacific find themselves caring for increasing numbers of ill relatives.

In households where this happens, incomes almost always decline, since HIV/AIDS disproportionately strikes young adults at the peak of their productive and earning powers. A study in Thailand's Chiang Mai province found that the foregone lifetime income of a deceased worker was

30 per cent higher when the person had died of AIDS than when they had died of non-HIV/AIDS-related causes (Pitayon *et al.* 1997).

In the same Chiang Mai study, HIV/AIDS-affected families reported spending an average of $1,000 in direct medical costs during the last year of life (*ibid.*). In Cambodia, expenditure was found to equal several times an extended family's annual income. In the rural parts of Cambodia, the high cost of medicine and the rural credit system combined to make HIV/AIDS a significant cause of landlessness (ESCAP 2002b).

In the Chiang Mai study, one-third of the households interviewed reported an average 48 per cent decrease in household consumption. The World Bank's analysis is that the death of an income-earner decreases household food consumption by 15 per cent (Topouzis and Hemrich 1997). This level of decrease potentially places other family members at risk of illness. HIV/AIDS is never only one death – it is multiple deaths.

The study undertaken by Pitayon *et al.* in Chiang Mai found that 60 per cent of the households with an AIDS death had used up their savings, 44 per cent had sold land, 42 per cent had reduced their food consumption, 28 per cent had sold a vehicle, and 11 per cent had borrowed money.

A gender analysis of the impact of HIV illness and death on household livelihoods highlights that women with lesser or no control over resources are the worst hit. The extent of this can be seen clearly in a study undertaken in Zimbabwe in 1999 by UNIFEM. The researchers of this study came up with the concept of the 'negative income shock' to describe the clinical condition of women in households affected by HIV – the impact of reaching a state of high expenditure and no income in a very short span of time, leaving them in a state of mental and physical shock. In the study, 77 per cent of persons experiencing this shock were women.

A wake-up call for Asia and the Pacific?

How does the Asia and Pacific region compare to Africa in terms of its ability to withstand the HIV/AIDS epidemic, and what lessons may be learnt from the African experience to help us prepare for the worst of the epidemic?

Social indicators

Compared to some of the African countries with mature HIV epidemics, for example Botswana, Zimbabwe, and South Africa, some countries in Asia – especially those in South Asia – are at a comparatively low starting point in terms of social indicators. Social indicators relate to: primary net enrolment ratios; GNP (gross national product) per capita; population with access to health services; population below the income poverty line of $2 per day. This is likely to constrain the countries' ability to respond meaningfully or with speed to the challenges of the HIV/AIDS epidemic.

Governance and political stability

Compared to Africa, the Asia and Pacific region has more political stability, which bodes well for its ability to manage and combat HIV/AIDS through government and donor responses. Although terrorism is a political concern in some countries of Asia, the political, social, and economic disaster of war has not created large numbers of displaced migrant populations, as has been the case in many countries of Africa. Most Asian and Pacific regions have effective systems of governance in place. These systems have the potential to generate local resources, and to demand accountability from policy makers and planners regarding the way development resources are channelled. Questions that the development community is already asking itself in hindsight for Africa could be relevant in relation to preventing crisis in Asia and the Pacific. They include:

- Could we have stopped the epidemic in Africa if we had invested prudently and strategically in reducing the incidence of sexually transmitted infections (STIs) and reproductive tract infections (RTIs) on the African continent? There is now ample evidence to show that the presence of these infections increases the chances of HIV transmission fivefold. The costs incurred by nations in preventing and curing these infections would have been a fraction of the costs incurred in treating HIV/AIDS.

- Could we have stopped the epidemic in some African countries if we had not believed that countries with high literacy rates would be less vulnerable to HIV/AIDS? For a number of years development workers believed in the view that education was perhaps the AIDS vaccine. It was as late as 1998 when the development indicators for some African countries began to depict the glaring contradictions of this view. For example, Zimbabwe, with a school enrolment rate of 84 per cent for girls and 89 per cent for boys, had an HIV prevalence rate of 26 per cent (UNDP 1998).

- Could we have stopped the HIV/AIDS epidemic in Africa by promoting the dual use of the condom (as a contraceptive, and a means for HIV/AIDS prevention) in time? In most countries, the condom has been seen by communities as a contraceptive alone, and was associated with family-planning programmes rather than programmes focusing on HIV/AIDS. Furthermore, as programmes on HIV/AIDS got progressively more and more compartmentalised, rather than being integrated into programmes on reproductive health, this misperception was exacerbated.

- Could we have stopped the epidemic in Africa if we had helped communities to 'unlearn' the myths and rituals around sexuality? The list of the myths and practices that have enshrouded human sexuality in different cultures is long.

These questions should be a wake-up call for us as we consider how to confront the pandemic in Asia and the Pacific.

Strategies to fight HIV/AIDS

In this section, I discuss some possible ways in which the impact of HIV/AIDS, and its spread, can be mitigated through policy responses.

Clearly, immediate implementation of *a comprehensive set of interventions* can avert a large number of future infections and reverse the likely course of the AIDS epidemic. A delayed response would significantly reduce the total benefits measured in terms of new infections prevented. For example, analyses suggest that a three-year delay in achieving full implementation of an expanded and comprehensive response would reduce by half the total number of new infections averted by 2010 (Stover *et al.* 2002).

Mainstreaming both gender and HIV into development

Mainstreaming gender and HIV into ongoing development projects in some key development sectors can be one of the most potent tools to speed the response to HIV/ AIDS. Mainstreaming gender and HIV into these sectors means climbing onto a horse that has already gathered momentum. Both working to promote equality between women and men, and working to prevent and treat HIV, require this approach.

This approach, however, requires a thorough understanding of the concepts of gender and of sexuality. An understanding of male and female sexual behaviour requires an awareness of how gender and sexuality are constructed by a complex interplay of social, cultural, and economic forces that affect the distribution of power. Mainstreaming gender and HIV into development programmes is, therefore, not about targeting women. It is not a game of numbers to show how many men participated as compared to how many women; rather, it is about understanding power relations between the sexes, about understanding why and how the HIV epidemic affects women and men differently, and about understanding the ways in which women and men cope. This approach necessitates the analysis of gender stereotypes and the exploration of ways to reduce inequalities between men and women. Ultimately, this enhances understanding of the obstacles to HIV prevention and coping, and provides direction for potential solutions to cope better with the epidemic.

Addressing HIV/AIDS through good governance

Development workers who are concerned with the agenda of good governance should also consider HIV/AIDS in their work. Today, in most countries of Asia and the Pacific, as in Africa, the gap between policy and implementation can be seen in the poor quality of life of the people who are meant to benefit from HIV-related policies and resource allocations. The most strategically placed agency of change that works with all sectors of the government is undoubtedly the National Audit. The Audit office is the only agency with the mandate to examine the gap between policy statements and implementation, and scrutinise the reasons for it. The National Audit is an influential process that is taken notice of by the highest policy-making and implementation bodies. The report of the Comptroller and Auditor General is presented to the head of state, is placed on the floor of the legislature for discussion, and is the basis of political questioning of the executive. In addition it has the potential to influence the public discourse through media. The law has little power to enforce policies, but developing the capacities of the Audit to analyse gender and HIV issues, and to bring these into sharp focus, is essential. In countries in which civil society is weak, ministries responsible for non-implementation of policy can be held accountable to see that people's entitlements to health care and other services are respected.

Hence, audits can potentially play a key role in enhancing the processes of good governance around HIV/AIDS prevention, and responses to people infected and affected by HIV/AIDS. Mainstreaming HIV in all sectors of development by working with the office of the Comptroller and Auditor General is worth considering as a strategy for Asian and Pacific countries.

Conclusion

African experience of the pandemic needs to inform discussions of the impact of HIV in Asia and the Pacific. Women in Africa today – and particularly younger women – are at risk of infection because of their inability to negotiate the terms on which they have sex. At the same time, the escalating costs of caring for those with the virus mean increasing demands on women's unpaid labour. In Asia as in Africa, we will witness a feminisation of the pandemic, and also assaults on women's dignity and rights, unless we sit up and take notice of unequal power between women and men. We also need to help women who are bearing the main burden of caring for those with HIV. Will the position and condition of women worsen in Asia and the Pacific due to HIV, or will systems of governance, in partnership with civil society, create the means for women and men to live, cope, and die with dignity?

Within civil society, there is courageous work being done by NGOs. Ashok, who runs the Humsafar Trust in Mumbai, is organising men who have sex with men, making them aware of the risks of bisexuality and instilling in them the principles of gender and power relations. He told me: 'We need to engage communities in newer discourses around sexual orientation.' In Cambodia, Aun is living positively with her second husband who is also HIV-positive, and they are both working with a support group for people living with AIDS. They both feel wanted and valued. The work they do is important. The task for development workers in countries where the epidemic is still young is to transform this fragmented energy into a holistic force – a force that moves from questioning deep-rooted stereotypical approaches, to building a body of information that is grounded in reality, and is based on lived experience. Only then will the agencies of change be able to re-engineer development in this era of HIV/AIDS.

This article was originally published in Gender & Development, *volume 14, number 1, March 2006.*

References

ESCAP (2002a) *HIV/AIDS and Poverty – The Impact of HIV/AIDS in the ESCAP Region*, Bangkok: United Nations Economic and Social Commission for Asia and the Pacific (ESCAP).

ESCAP (2002b) *Protecting Marginalised Groups during Economic Downturns: Lessons from the Asian Experience*, Bangkok: United Nations Economic and Social Commission for Asia and the Pacific (ESCAP).

ESCAP/UNDCP/UNAIDS (2001) *Injecting Drug Use and HIV Vulnerability – Choices and Consequences in Asia and the Pacific*, Bangkok: United Nations Economic and Social Commission for Asia and the Pacific (ESCAP).

Monitoring the AIDS Pandemic (2001) *The Status and Trends of HIV/AIDS/STI Epidemics in Asia and the Pacific*, United States Bureau of the Census Provisional Report 4 October 2001, Melbourne, Australia.

National AIDS Control Organization, Ministry of Health and Family Welfare, Government of India (2001) *Behavioural Surveillance Survey (BSS) 2001 Projections for HIV/AIDS in Thailand 2001–2020*, Division of AIDS, Department of Communicable Disease Control, Ministry of Public Health, Government of Thailand.

Pitayon, S., S. Kongsin, and W. Jangareon (1997) 'The economic impact of HIV/AIDS mortality on households in Thailand', in D. Bloom (ed.) *The Economics of HIV/AIDS*, Calcutta/Chennai/Mumbai: Oxford University Press.

Sarkar, S. (2003) 'Accelerating the Momentum in the Fight against HIV/AIDS in South Asia', paper presented at a high-level conference organised by UNICEF in Kathmandu, Nepal, 3–4 February 2003.

Shalini, B. (2000) *Impact of HIV/AIDS on Women in Households*, a report of indicative research undertaken on 30 households, Mumbai, India: Tata Institute of Social Sciences (TISS).

Stover, J. *et al.* (2002) 'Can we reverse the HIV/AIDS epidemic with an Expanded Response?', *The Lancet* 360(9326): 76.

Topouzis, D. and G. Hemrich (1997) *The Implications of HIV/AIDS for Rural Development – Policy and Programming*, New York: HIV and Development Programme, United Nations Development Programme (UNDP).

UNAIDS (2004) *2004 Report on the Global AIDS Epidemic: 4th Global Report*, Geneva: UNAIDS.

UNDP (1996) *Human Development Report*, New York: Oxford University Press.

UNDP (1998) *Human Development Report*, New York: Oxford University Press.

UNIFEM (2002) *The Socio-Economic Impact of HIV/AIDS in Vietnam Advocacy Folder Entitled 'Community Base Research on the Gender Dimensions of HIV/AIDS – Summary of Findings'*, New York: United Nations Development Fund For Women.

Notes

1 The tumbling of the Asian tigers relates to the depression in the Asian economy (especially in the countries of South-East Asia) in the last three years of the 1990s. The economic growth of the early nineties in these countries was a result of fast marketisation of these economies, which encouraged heavy investments by multi-national corporations (MNCs) without adequate safeguards to ensure that the capital generated would be used to promote equity and growth within the countries. As a result when the MNCs withdrew their capital, these economies crumpled.

2 'Progress' here refers to progress made on three indicators of human development – life expectancy, literacy, and per capita income. This progress was measured over 30 years, 1960–1990, by the UNDP Human Development Report of 1990 written by Mahbub-ul-Huq.

5 Safe motherhood in the time of AIDS: the illusion of reproductive 'choice'

Carolyn Baylies

'It's frightening to think that I am sitting at home while the "old man" might be wandering, moving from woman to woman to end up bringing HIV/AIDS home to me. I feel that I would even have no children at all so as not to be exposed to the risk of being HIV infected. The only "medicine" is to remain celibate and avoid getting married because that is the most likely situation in which a woman will get infected, considering unfaithful husbands.'

'If I suspected I were HIV-positive, I would stop having children because this would hasten my death. If I suspected my husband was promiscuous I would definitely have no more children with him.'

The comments above reflect women's anxieties about child-bearing when the prevalence of HIV infection is high and suspicions are harboured about partners' sexual behaviour. They were collected in a study carried out in Zambia in 1995, on the impact of AIDS on households in Chipapa, south of Lusaka, and Minga, in the country's Eastern Province.[1]

Given the importance of child-bearing in many societies, and their own desire for children, women often face a stark dilemma. As Marge Berer and Sunanda Ray put it, 'Practising safer sex and trying to get pregnant are not possible at the same time, at least on fertile days, and it may take many months or years for a woman to complete her family' (Berer with Ray 1993, 77). Topouzis and du Guerny comment that, 'If, under certain epidemiological conditions, a woman runs a 25 per cent chance of HIV infection in order to conceive, it follows that if she wants four, five or six children, she runs a very high risk of contracting HIV' (Topouzis and du Guerny 1999, 13). Women repeatedly stare those risks in the face, sometimes preferring not to acknowledge them fully, but often deciding that the costs of forgoing having children are much greater than the potential costs of HIV infection. Both of the women quoted above already had children. Younger, childless women might be less prone to articulate such views so forcibly, or to act on them.

Dilemmas around bearing children are also faced by men, but they have greater immediacy for women, due to the unequal power relations which characterise intimate relationships between men and women. Men tend to have more sexual partners during their lifetime, and more extra-marital encounters. Marriage – and fertility within it – is crucial to many women's economic security. In any given setting, the way such dilemmas are constructed, understood, and worked through is affected by the accessibility of means of protection against infection and/or contraception, opportunities for women's economic autonomy, and the level of HIV prevalence. A woman's age, marital status, level of education, and child-bearing history also have a bearing on the extent to which HIV may jeopardise chances of 'normal' maternity.

Neglect of women during the AIDS epidemic

As the AIDS epidemic gathered momentum in the late 1980s and early 1990s, a number of writers began to speak out about the way women had been neglected by both the medical profession and those involved with HIV prevention. Where they had been taken into account, women tended to be depicted not so much as individuals in their own right, vulnerable to HIV or suffering from illness and needing support, but as responsible for transmitting HIV to innocent children or, in the guise of 'blameworthy' sex workers, to male clients (Patton 1993; Sherr 1993; Carovano 1991). Women continue today to be widely cast in the role of transmitters of the virus. The relative visibility of commercial sex workers has made them a ready target for interventions – and an attractive one, if promoting their safer behaviour allows men to continue to be sexually 'mobile'.

Pregnant women are an even more accessible group for targeting. Throughout the course of the epidemic, the basis for estimates of HIV prevalence in populations has been surveillance testing at ante-natal clinics. The increasing possibility of mother-to-child infections being prevented through medical means has added a compelling logic for pregnant women being tested for HIV on a more routine basis.[2]

Over time, HIV/AIDS prevention campaigns have been directed at women more generally, based on an assumption that women tend to be the guardians of their families' health. But there are limits to such strategies, as women are frequently ill-placed to ensure that prevention messages which call for a reduction in the number of sexual partners, or use of condoms, are put into practice (Hamlin and Reid 1991; Sherr 1996). Only recently has there been a more concerted shift towards targeting men, in recognition of the fact that they 'drive the epidemic' (Foreman 1999). Men are increasingly called on to be responsible (Rivers and Aggleton 1998; Cohen and Reid 1996), via a paternalistic version of moral guardianship of their families' health. In Thailand, for example, male clients have been targeted alongside sex workers, and urged not so much to give up their extra-marital pursuits, as to use condoms, so as to provide some protection not just for themselves (and, incidentally, for sex workers), but also for their wives and children.

However, despite the fact that the position of wives as innocent victims of AIDS has been increasingly highlighted, there is still a large gap between the health and welfare needs of women in the face of AIDS and the attention and protection they actually receive. Their situation can be further complicated, and their ability both to control their fertility and to achieve truly safe motherhood can be jeopardised, when approaches to family planning discourage married women from using condoms as contraception in favour of more effective, hormonal means. On the other hand, in situations in which sexual abstinence and condom-use are designated as the primary means of protection from AIDS, women who wish to have children are frequently left 'with no options at all' (Carovano 1991, 136).

Limits on women's ability to choose

If one considers societal norms about fertility, together with the agendas of family-planning organisations and AIDS-protection campaigns, one can see the dilemmas of women very clearly. The language of choice, preference, planning, and decision-making, often used by health providers, emphasises the reproductive rights that all should enjoy. But these terms often misrepresent what actually occurs. Their use obscures the complexity of a process of negotiating – or failing to negotiate – the nature of sexual activity, which is grounded in power relations, convention, the heat of the moment, and, sometimes, gender violence.

Both men and women may feel aggrieved that they have less control than they might like over fertility 'outcomes', but women typically have far less control than their partners, in spite of terminology which labels many contraceptives 'women-controlled' (Lutalo *et al.* 2000). Many couples do communicate about having children and about the number of children they would like to have, but as Wolff *et al.* (2000) demonstrate with reference to a study in Uganda, they often experience difficulty in talking about such issues, use unspoken or indirect cues, or frequently misinterpret their partner's preferences, with men having a greater tendency than women to underestimate their partner's desire to stop having children. Nor, when they discuss such issues, does this necessarily imply equal participation or joint decision-making (see also Bauni and Jarabi 2000). It may rather serve as a basis for men to enforce their preferences.

Women typically have even less control over their fertility when accessibility to contraceptives is limited, as is more likely to be the case in rural than urban areas, or where contraceptive use is discouraged by religious dictates. There are considerable differences between countries, reflecting in part the varying scope of national or voluntary-sector family-planning programmes. For example, in 1994, 43 per cent of women aged 20–49 in Zimbabwe reported that they were currently using 'any contraceptive method', while the figure in neighbouring Zambia in 1996 was just 23 per cent (Blanc and Way 1998; Central Statistical Office *et al.* 1997).

HIV protection within marriage

Across most of Africa and many other parts of the developing world, however, the majority of women do not use 'modern' means of contraception, or indeed any means (Blanc and Way 1998). This amounts to a substantial unmet need for effective fertility control. Many women similarly have limited ability to protect themselves from HIV, not least within marriage, and especially during its early years when families are being built. The power relations which operate in this context are not absolute, and vary from place to place and according to other factors, such as the level of education of partners. But they typically serve to put women at a disadvantage. In the mid-1990s in Zambia, 65 per cent of married women considered themselves to be at risk of getting AIDS, as against 54 per cent of those formerly married and 35 per cent of those never married. Almost all of those married women who considered themselves at moderate or great risk gave as their reason the fact that their husbands had multiple partners. Just under half of all married men also considered themselves at risk of AIDS, but for those who perceived the risk to be moderate or great, the primary reason was, once again, that they had multiple partners (Central Statistical Office *et al.* 1997).

Even when a woman strongly suspects that her partner may be carrying the HIV virus, she may feel that there is little she can do about it. In a focus group in Kenya, one woman despaired, 'There is nothing a woman can do, because it is the man who brought her to that house. She has to submit to her husband for sex. Women don't have any powers to decide on issues concerning sex' (Bauni and Jarabi 2000). Another woman concurred: 'You will be beaten if you refuse to have sex', while another stated: 'There is nothing I can do because he is my husband, and also, I don't know about what to use' (Bauni and Jarabi 2000). In the mid-1990s in Zambia, 24 per cent of currently married women said that there was either no way to protect themselves, or that they did not know of any way (Central Statistical Office *et al.* 1997). In the Eastern Province, the figure was 39 per cent. Marital relations may suffer in consequence of anxieties and suspicions around AIDS, and break-ups may occur. However, these seem more typically to involve men sending away wives, than women leaving their husbands (Carpenter *et al.* 1999). The fact that men often re-marry more quickly may account in part for higher rates of HIV among women who have experienced divorce and separation than women who are either single or married (Gregson *et al.* 1997, 1998; Kapiga *et al.* 1998).

When the facilitator in the Zambia research asked women in a focus group in Makungwa, a village near Minga in the Eastern Province, 'Have you ever heard of a condom?', some said they had, while others demurred. Only one woman said she had ever seen one. The women did not know where or how to get them. But it would matter little, they contended: 'Some, in fact most, men would not agree to use a condom.' And then one asked, 'Are there condoms for women?'

Condoms are a particular issue of contention, as they can be used for both family planning and protection from sexually transmitted infection, but are associated in much of Africa (as elsewhere) with casual encounters or commercial sex. This association has been strengthened by slogans used in AIDS-prevention campaigns in many African settings, which call for abstinence prior to marriage and fidelity within it, and for any lapses through pre-marital or extra-marital encounters to be protected through the use of condoms. In Thailand and India, there have been similarly strong messages promoting the use of condoms outside marriage. The success of such campaigns makes it increasingly difficult for the condom to be promoted as a viable means of protection in sex within marriage. Meanwhile, advocacy of its extra-marital use serves in turn to reinforce the expectation that men (in particular) are liable to stray, and to underline the distinction not so much between what is moral or immoral sex (although that certainly applies in the minds of some), but between reproductive and recreational sex, the former increasingly associated with marriage and the latter with extra-marital encounters. This presumes there to be a difference between men's and women's sexual needs, with men's needs dictating the nature of sexual encounters and the roles which partners assume within them (Holland *et al.* 1998; Giffin 1998).

Women often emphasise their difficulty in persuading their husbands to use condoms (Bauni and Jarabi 2000; Baylies *et al.* 2000), because a request of this nature implies lack of trust. It may be easier to negotiate the use of condoms as a contraceptive, which then offers a secondary benefit of protection from HIV. But once again, the association of condoms with illicit sex can make even this problematic. Both in attempting to secure protection and trying to control fertility, women may resort to secret means. As a woman in Bauni and Jarabi's (2000) study in Kenya commented, such methods were essential, given that husbands only wanted sex and had little interest in family planning. Female condoms would seem to be a possible remedy, since they are 'in the hands of' women. In practice, however, even if they were readily accessible, it is highly unlikely that female condoms could be used without the knowledge of partners; negotiation will still be required. Moreover, in the minds of some, the female condom connotes the same association with 'extra-marital' sex as does the male condom (Kaler 2001). Microbicides which are also spermicides – or which provide protection against infection while permitting pregnancy – may be more promising.

It is not through secretive agency that women are likely to gain genuine control, but rather through challenging and transforming the gender relations which put them at risk in the first place. Without this, and without a change in men's behaviour, the problem of reconciling desired fertility with protection will remain.

Fertility among women who are HIV-positive

Many women do not know whether they or their partners are HIV-positive, and often, with much imprecision, use their children's health as a marker of their own. The anxiety a woman feels may not necessarily impact on her child-bearing, but she may wish to hedge her bets by having fewer children (Baylies 2000; Gregson *et al.* 1997, 1998) or, as one woman in Minga, Zambia explained, by having them more quickly so that if she becomes ill she will already have completed her family. But what of the situation of those who wish to have children when they already know that they are living with HIV or AIDS?

The situation may have changed substantially for some women elsewhere over recent years. But in Zambia, where few women have access to technical means of conceiving safely or to medication which could prolong lives, there are strong views that HIV-positive women should not have children. As one woman in Chipapa, Zambia, said, 'I would not have any more children if I found that I was positive. What is the point when they will end up dying?' While it overestimates the probability of HIV transmission from a woman to her children, this is a view deeply felt and often repeated, sometimes supplemented with the rationale that the woman's health would deteriorate should she become pregnant and she would also die 'soon'. Such sentiments reflect strong feelings of guilt about children being brought into the world only to face a quick death, and a sensitivity to the costs borne by wider society, even if their lives are short.

Yet even where there is little or no access to new therapies, such is the combination of pressure on women to have children and their own desire to conceive that many women who are aware that they are HIV-positive continue to become pregnant, especially those who are younger or in new relationships (Ryder *et al.* 2000; Santos *et al.* 1998). In many cases this is a consequence of a deeply felt need. Reporting on a small study of 21 women in Côte d'Ivoire diagnosed as HIV-positive during pregnancy, Aka-Dago-Akribi *et al.* (1999) note that even though the women were 'warned' about the possible consequences, their desire for another child remained very strong, except among those who already had at least four. All six who had given birth to only one child wanted another, as did two-thirds of those with two or three children. Only four of the 21 were using condoms. A study of women living with HIV in France found those with African backgrounds more likely to express a desire for more children and to have a child after a positive diagnosis than Caucasian women (Bungener *et al.* 2000).

A larger study of HIV-positive women in Europe found a higher rate of abortions and lower birth rates among them than within the general population, but a greater chance of pregnancy among those younger and born outside Europe, underlining the extent to which reproductive behaviour is related to cultural and social attitudes (van Benthem *et al.* 2000).[3]

Earlier in the epidemic, Bury (1991, 47) noted that decisions about pregnancy taken by women who are living with HIV are determined by a range of factors other than their own health and that of the child. 'She may wish to have a baby as it may be the only creative thing she has ever done. Knowledge of her HIV status and the realisation that she may die soon may be added reasons for wanting to fulfil herself in some way before she dies, and to leave something of herself after she is gone.' Hepburn (1991, 62) commented along similar lines that while some would prefer not to risk the possibility of a child being infected with HIV, 'Others consider having a child so important that any level of risk would be acceptable', with cultural, moral, or religious factors exerting a strong influence over considerations about contraception or termination.

Women who become pregnant when they are aware of their HIV status may be exercising choice, and, in the relatively rare cases where technical means permit, may be able to do so while their partners remain safe from infection. Where drug therapies are available, they can also minimise the probability of HIV transmission to their children. In many cases, however, factors associated with the context in which women live mean there is no possibility of 'choice' or 'control' over fertility or its outcomes. Fear of abandonment may make women reluctant to inform partners of their HIV status, let alone change their fertility behaviour. In a study in Burkino Faso, for example, this anxiety lay behind the fact that fewer than one-third of women who had been diagnosed with HIV told their partners about the diagnosis (Issiaka *et al.* 2001; see also Keogh *et al.* 1994; Ryder *et al.* 1991; Aka-Dago-Aribi *et al.* 1999; Santos *et al.* 1998). Marriage or customary unions may be based on affection, but are typically also entered into and sustained for reasons of economic security, which become all the more pressing when women are pregnant, newly delivered, or have a number of young children.

Moreover, some pregnancies among women with HIV may result from pressure from their partners, even when women's partners are informed about their HIV status (Bungener *et al.* 2000). Among the 45 per cent of HIV-positive women studied by Keogh *et al.* (1994) who gave birth over a three-year follow-up period, slightly fewer than half of pregnancies were 'planned', with four of these having been wanted by the male partner only. Lutalo *et al.* (2000) suggest that the couples they studied in Uganda appeared motivated to have children largely in order to meet social obligations, despite risks of transmission, and speculate that this might reflect the patrilineal culture of the area. Although some were using contraception, fewer than half were using condoms. Similar instances of unprotected sex have been found in other studies (Hira *et al.* 1990; Keogh *et al.* 1994; Santos *et al.* 1998) of couples where one or both had been diagnosed with HIV, in some cases as a consequence of their partners' opposition to using protection.

However, this pattern is neither uniform nor universal. While a third of women in Keogh *et al.*'s study were not using condoms, many of the others were. Moreover, there is some evidence of condoms being used for protection, alongside negotiated attempts to conceive in as much safety as possible. Thus, Ryder *et al.* (2000) report on predominantly safe pregnancies among 24 couples (albeit involving one new HIV infection) where women tried to restrict instances of unprotected sex to times when they considered themselves most fertile. But this was a case involving a high level of support from research and medical teams, which is unavailable to most couples.

Particular problems for young, unmarried women

Particularly complicated dilemmas arise in respect of sexual relations among unmarried young people, not least because this is an area beyond the boundaries of what many regard as 'legitimate fertility' (Garenne *et al.* 2000). Data from health and demographic surveys conducted during the 1990s indicate that many – in some age groups most – young people in developing countries are not sexually active (Blanc and Way 1998) and a relatively small minority have multiple partners. Moreover, the age of sexual initiation is rising in many societies. However, the gap between age of sexual initiation and age at first marriage is increasing, marking not just the possibility of pregnancy but also the extent of potential danger of HIV infection where sex is unprotected (Blanc and Way 1998). Young women are especially susceptible to HIV infection, in consequence of physiological immaturity, higher susceptibility to other sexually trasmitted diseases (STDs), and vulnerability to non-consensual sex (UNAIDS 1999; Baden and Wach 1998).

Young people are often left in the lurch, targeted by AIDS-prevention campaigns exhorting them to abstain from sex, given incomplete sex education by schools, parents, or traditional educators, and largely excluded from family-planning campaigns (Baylies *et al.* 1999; Garenne *et al.* 2000). They inhabit a milieu of rapidly changing, contradictory sexual norms with mixed messages from parents, peers, and AIDS campaigners. Significantly, they are often left with limited access to means of either contraception or protection against HIV. Their first sexual encounters are almost always unprotected, and they are more likely than older people to experience contraceptive failure (Blanc and Way 1998).

For young women, choice in respect of both child-bearing and ensuring protection may be particularly problematic. Social pressures may bear heavily upon them, albeit in contradictory ways. Nyanzi *et al.* (2000) describe how tensions between traditional attitudes towards female chastity and modern notions of sexual freedom complicate the lives of adolescents in Uganda. Gage (1998) notes that, in several African societies, girls are under pressure on the one hand to avoid having children, and on the other to prove their fertility, whether to secure a relationship or to demonstrate themselves to be a desirable partner. Many young people are adopting protective practices, but this is less true of women than men, and, as Baggaley *et al.* (1997) show in their study of university students in Zambia, it is more likely to occur during casual encounters than with regular partners. Frequently, young people face the future with a high level of fatalism, adopting what appears to their parents to be a brazen attitude, but to their peers a sophisticated realism. They frequently misperceive risks and harbour false confidence about their safety. As Hulton *et al.* (2000) note in reference to a Uganda study, boys often see sex as natural and predominantly for pleasure, and pregnancy as accidental. Adolescent girls may contrive ingenious means of dealing with potential sexual partners, yet show reluctance to introduce condoms into their sexual negotiations, conceding when their partners reject protection on grounds that it hinders male pleasure (Nyanzi *et al.* 2000).

The possibility of more positive outcomes

The dilemmas facing women who wish to bear children in safety are many and multi-faceted. A few may choose to forgo the great satisfaction of having children. Some will be fortunate enough to secure responsible partners. But most will take risks with their lives, whether after weighing up the odds and deciding that the potential rewards are greater than the probable costs, or preferring to take a more fatalistic stance. However, once women have had one or two children, they may approach the future more cautiously.

There is evidence that some women (and some men) may consider limiting the size of their families, not just in the interests of their own and their partner's safety, but in order to maximise the welfare of their children (Baylies 2000). HIV/AIDS creates uncertainty about parents' ability to survive long enough to ensure their children's welfare. The fewer those children, the greater the chance that they might be reasonably well looked after by relatives. There is also evidence that some women are now choosing to leave husbands suspected of engaging in risky behaviour. In the Zambia research, a young woman in Chipapa, near Lusaka, who was living in her parents' home and looking after her small child, first answered a question about how the threat which HIV posed might affect her child-bearing behaviour by saying she was frightened of getting HIV, and if she felt her spouse was endangering her by being promiscuous, she would not only stop bearing his children, but promptly leave him. But then she elaborated, moving from the hypothetical to the intensely personal: 'In fact, I am divorced, because my ex-husband wanted to have two wives and brought in another woman. I am not interested in a polygamous marriage, and would sooner remain single than risk my life.'

The choice to leave a marriage is bound up with economic considerations, and is influenced by the number and age of the children. In some cases, older children are able to assist their mothers to ensure subsistence, especially in agricultural communities. In other cases, the fewer children a woman has, the more likely she is to be able to support her family as a lone parent. The mother of a young child in Zambia's Copperbelt explained to a research colleague how she had gone to stay with her mother at the time of the birth. On her return, she discovered that her husband had taken up with a girlfriend, who had been 'taken home for illegally sleeping with him'. He pleaded with his wife for forgiveness, whereupon she demanded that he have an HIV test. When he refused, she left him. 'It is better to be divorced now, when we have only one child, than when we have a lot of children,' she said. Her friend agreed, noting that many women who might otherwise wish to do so 'fail' to leave their husbands because they are concerned about the future of their children (Chabala, field notes, 25 February 1999). The more children they have, the greater their sense that their children's welfare depends on the material security which marriage affords.

In conclusion, sexual practices and identities, which contribute so fundamentally to a sense of cultural stability, often appear to be 'permanent and natural' (Herdt 1997, 8). Yet radical change is possible. HIV presents a challenge to sexual practices and identities, exposing their dangers. There is a certain intransigence in this area, and not a little fatalism; arguments of 'naturalness' and male 'need' prop up structures of inequitable power and privilege. Yet the sexual practices and identities of women and men are continuously undergoing change. The negative and positive potential of this change process is sharply illuminated in the face of AIDS. While young people are placed in particular danger, the greater autonomy they strive for can set the stage for a more considered approach to their future mutual survival. But perhaps the issue can be most forcefully addressed by the generation adjacent to them, and particularly by women who already have at least some children. If their husbands fail to behave 'responsibly', such women may determine that for their own safety and the ultimate welfare of their children, they must go their own way. But they must, in turn, do so responsibly. Of necessity, the HIV/AIDS epidemic forces a sober look at sexual practices and identities, and the power relations which inform them. It has brought some change – although admittedly also some return to older practices. But it will require not just change in behaviour, but much more fundamental change in the nature of gender relations if conceiving children is to be safe for both women and men in future, and for their offspring.

This article was originally published in Gender & Development, *volume 9, number 2, July 2001.*

References

Aka-Dago-Akribi, H., A. Desgrees du Lou, P. Msellati, R. Dossou, and C. Welffens-Ekra (1999) 'Issues surrounding reproductive choice for women living with HIV in Abidjan', *Reproductive Health Matters*, 7(13).

Baden, S. and H. Wach (1998) 'Gender, HIV/AIDS transmission, and impacts: a review of issues and evidence', *Bridge*, Report no. 47, Institute of Development Studies, University of Sussex, UK.

Baggaley, R., F. Drobniewski, A. Pozniak, D. Chipanta, M. Tembo, and P. Godfrey-Faussett (1997) 'Knowledge and attitudes to HIV and AIDS and sexual practices among university students in Lusaka, Zambia and London, England: are they so different?', *Journal of the Royal Society of Health*, 117(2): 88–94.

Bauni, E. and B. Jarabi (2000) 'Family planning and sexual behaviour in the era of HIV/AIDS: the case of Nakuru District, Kenya', *Studies in Family Planning* 31(1): 69–80.

Baylies, C. (2000) 'The impact of HIV on family size preference in Zambia', *Reproductive Health Matters*, 8(15).

Baylies, C., J. Bujra, *et al.* (1999) 'Rebels at risk, young women and the shadow of AIDS', in C. Becker, J.-P. Dozon, C. Obbo, and M. Toure (eds.), *Experiencing and Understanding AIDS in Africa*, Dakar/ Paris: Codesria/Editions Karthala/IRD.

Baylies, C., J. Bujra, and the Gender and AIDS Group (2000) *AIDS, Sexuality and Gender in Africa: Collective Strategies for Protection Against AIDS in Tanzania and Zambia*, London: Routledge.

Berer, M. with S. Ray (1993) *Women and HIV/AIDS, An International Resource Book*, London: Pandora.

Bergenstrom, A. and L. Sherr (2000) 'A review of HIV testing policies and procedures for pregnant women in public maternity units of Porto Alegre, Rio Grande do Sul, Brazil', *AIDS Care*, 12(2): 177–86.

Blanc, A. and A. Way (1998) 'Sexual behaviour and contraceptive knowledge and use among adolescents in developing countries', *Studies in Family Planning*, 29(2): 106–16.

Bungener, C., N. Marchand-Gonod, and R. Jouvent (2000) 'African and European HIV-positive women: psychological and psychosocial differences', *AIDS Care*, 17(5): 541–8.

Bury, J. (1991) 'Pregnancy, Heterosexual Transmission and Contraception', in Bury, Morrison, and McLachlan (eds.), *Working With Women and AIDS*, London: Routledge.

Carovano, K. (1991) 'More than mothers and whores: redefining the AIDS prevention needs of women', *International Journal of Health Services*, 21(1): 131–42.

Carpenter, L., A. Kamali, A. Ruberantwari, S. Malamba, and A. Whitworth (1999) 'Rates of HIV-1 transmission within marriage in rural Uganda in relation to the HIV sero-status of the partners', *AIDS*, 13: 1083–9.

Central Statistical Office [Zambia], Ministry of Health, and Macro International, Inc. (1997) *Zambia Demographic and Health Survey 1996*, Calverton MD: Central Statistical Office and Macro International, Inc.

Cohen, D. and E. Reid (1996) 'The Vulnerability of Women: is this a Useful Construct for Policy and Programming?', Issues Paper no. 28, New York: UNDP HIV and Development Programme.

Foreman, M. (ed.) (1999) *AIDS and Men, Taking Risks or Taking Responsibility?* London: Panos/Zed Books.

Gage, A. (1998) 'Sexual activity and contraceptive use: the components of the decision-making process', *Studies in Family Planning*, 29(2): 154–66.

Garenne, M., S. Tollman, and K. Kahn (2000) 'Premarital fertility in rural South Africa: a challenge to existing population policy', *Studies in Family Planning*, 31(1): 47–54.

Giffin, K. (1998) 'Beyond empowerment: heterosexualities and the prevention of AIDS', *Social Science and Medicine*, 46(2): 151–6.

Gregson, S., *et al.* (1997) 'HIV and fertility change in rural Zimbabwe', *Health Transition Review*, 7(Supp. 2): 89–112.

Gregson, S., *et al.* (1998) 'Is there evidence for behaviour change in response to AIDS in rural Zimbabwe?', *Social Science and Medicine*, 46(3): 321–30.

Hamlin, J. and E. Reid (1991), 'Women, the HIV Epidemic and Human Rights: a Tragic Imperative', Issues Paper no. 8, New York: UNDP HIV and Development Programme.

Hepburn, M. (1991) 'Pregnancy and HIV, screening, counselling and services', in J. Bury, V. Morrison, and S. McLachlan (eds.), *Working with Women with AIDS*, London: Routledge.

Herdt, G. (1997) 'Sexual cultures and population movement: implications for AIDS/STDs', in G. Herdt (ed.), *Sexual Cultures and Migration in the Era of AIDS, Anthropological and Demographic Perspectives*, Oxford: Oxford University Press.

Hira, S., G. Mangrola, C. Mwale, C. Chintu, *et al.* (1990) 'Apparent vertical transmission of human immunodeficiency virus type 1 by breastfeeding in Zambia', *Journal of Paediatrics*, 117(3): 421–4.

Holland, J., C. Ramazanoglu, S. Sharpe, and R. Thompson (1998) *The Male in the Head, Young People, Heterosexuality and Power*, London: Tufnell Press.

Hulton, L., R. Cullen, and S. Khalokho (2000) 'Perceptions of risk of sexual activity and their consequences among Ugandan adolescents', *Studies in Family Planning*, 31(1): 35–46.

Issiaka, S., M. Cartoux, O. Ky-Zerbo, S. Tiendrebeogo, N. Meda, F. Daris, and P. Van de Perre, for the Ditrame Study Group (2001) 'Living with HIV: women's experience in Burkina Faso, West Africa', *AIDS Care*, 13(1): 123–8.

Kaler, A. (2001) '"It's some kind of women's empowerment": the ambiguity of the female condom as a marker of female empowerment', *Social Science and Medicine*, 53(5): 783–96.

Keogh, P., S. Allen, C. Almedal, and B. Temahagili (1994) 'The Social Impact of HIV Infection on Women in Kigali, Rwanda: a Prospective Study', *Social Science and Medicine*, 38(8): 1047–53.

Lutalo, T., M. Kidugavu, M. Wawer, D. Serwadda, Zabin, and R. Gray (2000) 'Trends and determinants of contraceptive use in Rakai District, Uganda 1995–98', *Studies in Family Planning*, 31(3): 217–27.

Nyanzi. S., R. Pool, and J. Kinsman (2000) 'The negotiation of sexual relationships among school pupils in south-western Uganda', *AIDS Care*, 13(1): 83–98.

Patton, C. (1993) '"With champagne and roses": women at risk from/in AIDS discourse', in C. Squire (ed.), *Women and AIDS, Psychological Perspectives*, London: Sage Publications.

Rivers, K. and P. Aggleton (1998) 'Men and the HIV Epidemic', New York: UNDP HIV and Development Programme.

Ryder, R.W., *et al.* (1991) 'Fertility rates in 238 HIV-1-seropositive women in Zaire followed for 3 years post-partum', *AIDS*, 5(12): 1521–7.

Ryder, R., C. Kamenga, M. Jingu, N. Mbuyi, and F. Behets (2000) 'Pregnancy and HIV-1 incidence in 178 married couples with discordant HIV-1 serostatus: additonal experience at an HIV-1 counselling centre in the Democratic Republic of Congo', *Tropical Medicine and International Health*, 5(7): 482–7.

Santos, N., E. Ventura-Filipe, and V. Palva (1998) 'HIV positive women, reproduction and sexuality in Sao Paulo, Brazil', *Reproductive Health Matters*, 6(12).

Sherr, L. (1993) 'HIV testing in pregnancy', in C. Squire (ed.), *Women and AIDS, Psychological Perspectives*, London: Sage Publications.

Sherr, L. (1996) 'Tomorrow's era: gender, psychology and HIV infection', in L. Sherr, C. Hankins, and L. Bennett (eds.), *AIDS as a Gender Issue, Psychological Perspectives*, London: Taylor & Francis.

Topouzis, D. and J. du Guerny (1999) 'Sustainable Agricultural/Rural Development and Vulnerability to the AIDS Epidemic', New York: FAO and UNAIDS, UNAIDS Best Practice Collection.

UNAIDS (1999) 'Differences in HIV spread in four sub-Saharan African cities, summary of the multi-site study', *UNAIDS Fact Sheet*, New York: UNAIDS.

van Benthem, B., I. de Vincenzi, M.-C. Delmas, C. Larsen, A. van den Hoek, M. Prins, and the European Study on the Natural History of HIV Infection in Women (2000) 'Pregnancies before and after HIV diagnosis in a European cohort of HIV-infected women', *AIDS*, 14: 2171–8.

Wolff, B., A. Blanc, and J. Ssekamatte-Ssebuliba (2000) 'The role of couple negotiation in unmet need for contraception and the decision to stop childbearing in Uganda', *Studies in Family Planning*, 31(2): 124–37.

Notes

1 The project involved small surveys, each with 150 participants, focus-group discussions, and in-depth interviews with a sub-set of the initial sample. The study was funded under the UK Government's Overseas Development Administration's (now Department for International Development) Links between Population and the Environment Research Programme. Among those involved in the research and its administration deserving particular mention are Veronica Manda, Mbozi Haimbe, Oliver Saasa, Beatrice Liatto-Katundu, Mary Zulu, Epiphano Phiri, Bornwell Maluluka, Edwin Cheelo, and Melanie Ndzinga.

2 While the primary objective of such testing is prevention of paediatric AIDS, in countries where wealth and political will exists, women found to be living with HIV infection may enjoy a secondary, fortuitous benefit via access to anti-retroviral drugs. This is not only the case for women in Europe and North America, but also in countries such as Brazil (see Bergenstrom and Sherr 2000; Santos *et al.* 1998).

3 The studies by Bungener *et al.* (2000) and van Benthem *et al.* (2000) were conducted in the mid-1990s. It is possible that the increased life expectancy that anti-retroviral regimes offer will alter HIV-positive women's calculations about having children, offering hope for more 'normal' maternity. But there is insufficient data to know how far this will be the case.

Part II
Rethinking 'our' attitudes to 'others'' realities

6 Diversifying gender: male to female transgender identities and HIV/AIDS programming in Phnom Penh, Cambodia

Barbara Earth

Cambodia's approach to HIV prevention is a good example of what is known as the 'behaviour change' model. Measures have overwhelmingly focused on increasing condom use: awareness-raising about condoms, increasing access to condoms, enacting laws that require 100 per cent condom use in sex establishments, training women sex workers to use condoms, and ensuring brothel owners' and police support. The emphasis on condom use has been reinforced through various media, including television, radio, newspapers, billboards, and other print media. Though these interventions have reduced the total number of infections, they have focused only on heterosexuals. Sexual minorities have not been targeted for any government HIV interventions, and there have not been any policy statements referring to them (MWVA 2003; NAA 2001).

In contrast, HIV/AIDS researchers in Asian contexts commonly remark on the array of gender identities they find. De Lind van Wijngaarden (1999), for example, found six different gender identities among male (*sic*) sex workers he studied in Chiang Mai, Thailand. Research suggests that sexualities diversify as an aspect of globalisation, due to the imposition of broadly similar economic and political policies, and the increasing influence of the Western media. The widespread introduction of Western sexual identity labels into non-Western societies has resulted in a merging of traditional sexualities with Western ones, to create hybrid identities (Altman 1995).

De Lind van Wijngaarden (1999) and Wichayanee (2006) further believe that the globalisation of the sex industry has also expanded sexual practices, sexualities, and identities worldwide.

Sexual diversities in Cambodia became visible to me personally in the course of a larger study of gender and HIV/AIDS in Phnom Penh (Earth 2005). That study interviewed various stakeholders including people living with HIV/AIDS, to understand the gendered aspects and limitations of HIV/AIDS prevention and care as currently practised; and to address the gaps in a city-wide action plan that was subsequently developed with nine government and NGO stakeholders. In the course of this work, several NGOs were found to be working with 'men who have sex with men' (this unsatisfactory term will be unpacked later in this article). These organisations were the USAID-funded NGO Family Health International (FHI), and two local NGOs, the Khmer HIV/AIDS NGO Alliance (KHANA) and the Urban Sector Group (USG). In my research, I interviewed staff of these organisations and members of their constituencies, and observed interactions at several cruising[1] places. Attending four conferences and meetings concerned with gender and sexuality in Asia then deepened the insights I gained from this experience.

Diverse genders and sexualities in Cambodia

South-East Asians understand gender and sexuality in terms less rigid than the Western categories of 'female' and 'male'.[2] In Thailand, for example, gender, sex, and sexuality are not distinct, but are merged into an integrated concept of who a person is. *Kathoey* was traditionally recognised as a third sex/gender. The term denoted either males or females whose bodies had characteristics of the other sex, or who exhibited behaviour that deviated from dominant gender norms (Jackson and Sullivan 1999). However, the term *kathoey* is now used almost exclusively to refer to those who have been raised as males (defined according to outer genitalia) who have a transgender[3] identity (Jackson and Sullivan 1999, 4), most often expressed in cross-dressing – that is, dressing as women (Brummelhuis 1999). The term *kteuy* denotes the same meaning in traditional Khmer society (personal communication, Phong Tan, 21 September 2005). A *kteuy* is not a man in the conventional sense, but is rather intermediate, a kind of woman, who has relations with men.

Other non-normative sexualities are also present. Same-sex activity among boys and men in Cambodian society has been commonplace and tolerated (Tarr 1996), though 'homosexual' is not a Cambodian concept. Heterosexual-identified male sex workers may sell sex to either men or women; these are men and are quite different from *kteuy*. Though male and female are the dominant genders, it is recognised that others exist, among whom are 'short hairs' and 'long hairs'.

'Short hairs' (Sak klay)

These people are also called *Pros saat* (handsome man). They identify themselves as men who have sex with men. These men may appear more feminine than the norm, but dress and identify as men, and are usually married. They wear their hair short like other men, and easily blend into the dominant society. Wives of 'short hairs' do not know the truth about their husbands.

Only a few 'short hairs' have sex only with men (interview, Men's Health Cambodia, 1 October 2004). Thus a lack of awareness among this sub-group makes not only themselves, but also their unknowing wives, very vulnerable to HIV. As part of the research, I accompanied a fieldworker known as 'Mom' on his nightly beat in a city park. A gaunt young man, whom Mom identified as a prostitute, told me that he did not think condoms were always necessary. It was obvious that his and his clients' risk was high, as business was brisk. Every night, hundreds of men meet at this venue alone. Mom said that awareness was higher than it had previously been, but that safe sex was not always practised (field notes, 1 October 2004). I observed that condoms were not available at the park, nor did outreach workers distribute them.

As stated earlier, 'short hairs' use the term 'men who have sex with men' to refer to themselves, and it seems to fit them, as they are men who have no outward characteristics that set them apart from mainstream heterosexual society. Of approximately 500 'short hairs' in Phnom Penh, about half identify with the organisation Men's Health Cambodia (MHC) for some sense of community with others of their kind. MHC works non-confrontationally for the acceptance of men who have sex with men in Cambodian society. It is a project funded by FHI, aiming to raise awareness on the need for condom use among 'short hairs' and their partners.

To reach this group, MHC has adopted the Men Helping Men model implemented in Thailand, in which fieldworkers (who are 'short hairs' themselves) walk particular 'beats' in cruising places used by men for sexual encounters, and disseminate information on safe sex. This development is significant, as historically these men have been invisible. Visits to MHC's storefront office in a fashionable area reveal a mostly young crowd, with increasing numbers of new faces, averaging 25 or more visitors per night (30 September 2004; 27 March 2005; 28 May 2005). Some 50 members were estimated to be HIV-positive (Mao Kimrun, 28 May 2005).

'Short hairs' adopt an assimilationist approach towards the wider society. They mingle easily with people from neighbouring shops during the nightly open hours at the MHC drop-in centre. They may dress up as *Srei Sros* (literally, 'charming girls') for parties, but do not cross-dress in public. An informant said that some 'short hairs' may psychologically be 'long hairs' (discussed in the next section), but they cut their hair short in order to 'pass' in society (Tun Samphy, 29 March 2005).

'Long hairs' (Srei Sros [*charming girls*])

Another non-normative sub-group in Cambodia is more obviously at odds with gender norms. They are transgender persons who identify as women, dress and act as women, and wear their hair long. 'Long hairs' may refer to themselves as *kteuy* but may consider it insulting to be described as such by others. 'Transwomen' is not a term they use, but may emerge as appropriate.

Previous studies have included them in the category of men who have sex with men, but this is an inaccurate use of terminology, because *Srei Sros* do not themselves identify as men. Rather, they refer to themselves as women, and reconfirm their identities every day by dressing and going out as women. Psychologically, *Srei Sros* are women, and they want to marry real men. They love men as heterosexual women do. They only sell sex to men (Tun Samphy, 29 March 2005). *Srei Sros*, because they radically transgress norms, suffer more discrimination in society than do 'short hairs'.

A 2004 census estimated 400 Srei Sros to be in Phnom Penh. Through USG, I met three of them, aged 28, 37, and 35. Though they were raised as boys, they feel themselves to be women, and have been living as women for many years. One of them began dressing as a girl at the age of ten. They use hormones to develop their breasts, but have not had surgery[4] (field notes, 16 June 2005). Because Cambodian society insists on at least a facade of heterosexuality, it is not possible for them to be settled in a sexual relationship. They sell sex both as a way of having their sexuality and as a livelihood. Selling sex is also proof of their womanhood. Around 5pm, they get dressed and go to meet clients in one of several outdoor places. They wear long skirts and behave modestly, as good Cambodian women should (observed at Wat Botom Park). Their clients are 'real men' (discussed later in this article) who range in age and marital status (the young ones not being married yet). The time they spend with a client may be one hour, half an hour, or all night, depending on how they feel about each other. They average two to three clients per night. Being older now, it is not as easy to get clients as it used to be when they were young (field notes, 16 June 2005).

Srei Sros are very vulnerable. Their deviation from gender norms and normal heterosexuality may arouse the rage of 'real men', who try to enforce norms through violence. Sometimes *Srei Sros* are subject to abuse from clients. Like other women, they are likely to have little power to negotiate safe sex. One of my informants is HIV-positive, and shares a room with a friend so that they can help and support each other.

Srei Sros have only themselves to rely on. Yet, their way of life is profoundly radical. (This is probably possible in contemporary Cambodia because *kteuy* have always existed openly.) Being true to one's identity amounts to active resistance against oppressive norms, lived resolutely every day. However, 'long hairs' do not have a sense of community. There is no drop-in centre for them from which to develop a community, and there is no activist tradition in Cambodia from which to draw lessons.

Rather, *Srei Sros* have personal friendships among themselves, and may maintain good relations with neighbours. Rich *Srei Sros* strive for artistic or commercial success to gain acceptance.

Cambodian *Srei Sros* may migrate to Thailand in search of better fortunes, but life is not easy for them in Thailand either. Because of historical tensions between the countries, Cambodian *Srei Sros* may be abused or raped in Thailand, and eight out of ten reportedly come back HIV-positive (personal communication, Tun Samphy, Program Coordinator of Sex Workers' Education for AIDS Reduction, USG, 29 March 2005).

'Real men' (Boroh pith brakat [*masculine man*])

The 'long hairs' and 'short hairs' comprise distinct gender groupings, but the objects of their desires are the same: 'real men'. Very little is known about the range of sexuality among real men, because they shun researchers (Catalla *et al.* 2003). Real men appear to be, and are considered to be, heterosexual, even though many are not heterosexual in the strictly literal sense. Though some real men have sex only with women, other real men may have sex with a range of different kinds of partners. These men hide their lifestyles and do not identify themselves as different, as they may have important jobs and cannot risk being known. They are, or will be, married conventionally to women.

Some real men sell sex, either to men or to women. As with women sex workers, it is their source of income, and is not related to their own sexual preference(s). Female clients do exist: during the course of walking the Wat Botom Park beat with my informant, 'Mom', I observed two women out of a sea of men and was informed that these women were there for sex, as was everyone else. Along the beat, I observed hundreds of men cruising, most of them real men. Mom introduced me to real men from high-level ministry offices who came in conspicuous, expensive cars. One of them smiled broadly as we exchanged greetings, his large diamond ring flashing in the darkness (field notes, 30 September 2004); however, interviewing was out of the question.

Some real men are violently prejudiced against non-normative men and transwomen, and may attack or rape them. This tendency was noted by (former) King Norodom Sihanouk who stated that real men (not sexual minorities) are the source of violence in society (personal communication, Mao Kimrun, Director of MHC, 1 October 2004).

Real men are the largest and most ambiguous identity category. When research does investigate and uncover the variations hidden within this category, we can imagine many diversities emerging. There are also constellations of female, and female-to-male, transgender sexualities, which are currently hidden. However, they would comprise another world altogether. Figure 1 gives a sense of how the various groups described here form part of the 'galaxy' of genders/sexualities and sexual networks in Phnom Penh.

In the next section, I examine the impact of HIV strategies that confine their understandings of gender to an analysis of heterosexual gender relations, in light of the complex realities of sexuality discussed here.

Figure 1: Some known sexual diversities in Phnom Penh with some known sexual networks

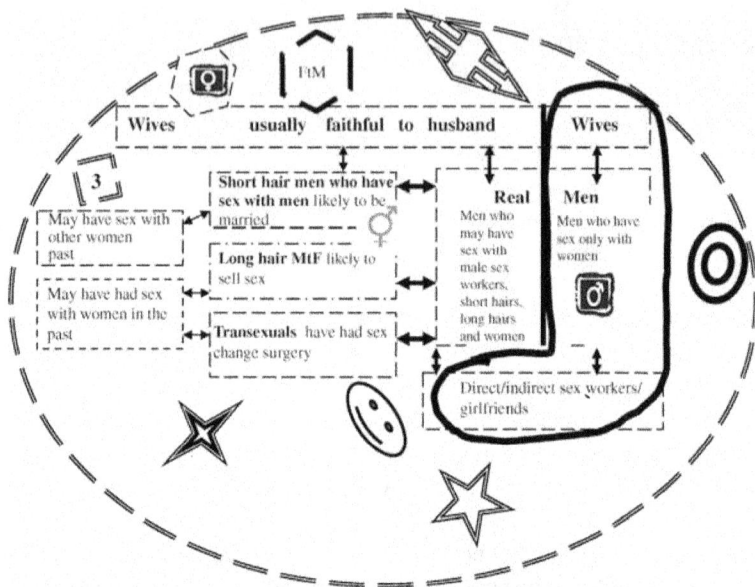

Circled components have been the sole focus of government HIV-prevention activities, leaving marginal groups vulnerable and likely to bridge HIV to other sectors. The shapes represent infinitely more queer possibilities. The figure should be imagined in multi-dimensional motion.

The impact of 'gender-blind' HIV strategies on marginalised groups

It can be seen from the above discussion that HIV-prevention strategies cannot focus on heterosexual people only. In reality, there are many genders/sexualities. HIV research has brought to light very different identities, contextual realities, and hence very different needs. HIV strategies need to take these into account, and to use the terms that individuals themselves use to identify themselves.

Because non-normative groups have been overlooked in HIV-prevention campaigns, they may not know how vulnerable they are. They may think that their sexual activities are safe, in contrast to sex between men and women, which prevention campaigns always link to condom use. The government's approach to HIV can have a harmful effect on both 'short hairs', men who have sex with men, and 'long hairs', *Srei Sros*. Bias towards heterosexual norms (which I argue is a type of gender bias) is the only explanation for such oversight on the part of the government, which has a duty to protect the health of all citizens.

A study by Girault et al. (2002) revealed that of 206 men who have sex with men (mostly male sex workers), 14.4 per cent had HIV. Some of my informants thought it impossible to know how many men who have sex with men are HIV-positive, because there is no budget for research, and no way to know the sexual identity or sexual activities of men (group interview, MHC, 1 October 2004). Another informant asserted that HIV is increasing among the *Srei Sros* she works with, estimating their HIV prevalence to be 20–30 per cent (Pak Kim San, Khmer Development of Freedom Organization, 9 August 2004).

By definition, male sex workers have sexual relations with more than one partner. In Girault et al.'s (2002) study, of the 206 men who reported selling sex or having sex with men, many also reported having sex with women. The respondents used condoms less frequently than direct (i.e. brothel-based) female sex workers, and far less consistently than other groups of high-risk men (Girault et al. 2002). The sexual networking patterns and the lack of safe-sex consciousness found among these men, suggest they are putting themselves, their clients, and their non-commercial partners, at high risk.

These finding support Mann and Tarantola's (1998) view that HIV/AIDS has a way of marking social inequality. Vulnerability entrenches itself among excluded groups, where HIV/AIDS remains intransigent. In Cambodia, the dominant understanding of 'gender' has excluded the most marginal people and thus increased their vulnerability to HIV.

Understanding the implications for political action

All development workers need to understand the very real political implications of our choices about the terminology we use, and the ways we classify the people with whom we work. What needs to change?

Changing vocabulary

A vocabulary has been introduced by the international HIV/AIDS sector that perpetuates an inaccurate picture of gender and sexual relations in the Cambodian context. The use of the term "men who have sex with men" is perhaps the most problematic. The definition by Girault et al. (2002) reveals several problems with the term: 'The term "men who have sex with men" refers to biological males who engage in sex with other biological males, irrespective of their motivation for their sexual behaviour and irrespective of their self-identification and even irrespective of whether they regard themselves as "men"' (Girault et al. 2002, 1).

Like most of us, Girault et al. apply the term naively. It has been scientifically established that 'biological male' is not a discrete or self-evident category. Throughout time and place, there have been people whose bodies have not conformed to the two categories, 'biological male' and 'biological female'. Sex may be ambiguous at birth or later. Many people develop primary or secondary sex characteristics that do not fit neat definitions of male or female (Koyama 2003). In North America, it is estimated that approximately 1 in 1,500 to 1 in 2,000 births require consultation with a specialist in sex differentiation. Many more people than that are born with subtler forms of sex anatomy variations, some of which do not show up until later in life (ISNA n.d.).

Further, naming people in particular ways, who do not want to be so named, certainly implies a degree of arrogance. According to Phong Tan (personal communication, 21 September 2005), the widespread usage of Western terms may force their adoption by gender-variant people, but inside, these individuals still think of themselves as *kteuy*. It is no surprise that the term 'men who have sex with men' is widely objected to, yet it persists.

Finally, the Girault *et al.* study reported aggregated results from all their respondents, labeling them as 'men who have sex with men'. This creates more confusion than clarification. A *kteuy* self-identifies not as a real man, but is, rather, a kind of woman who has relations with men; thus a *kteuy* is not 'homosexual'. It is clear that gender-variant people are not a single group, but a multiplicity of individuals/ groups with distinct psychologies. Male sex workers, who consider themselves heterosexual men, and who sell sex to either men or women, are located quite differently from *kteuy*, and both are distinct from effeminate men. Men who have sex with members of the above groups are also correspondingly different.

Terminology has direct implications for HIV/AIDS policy and programming. Just as an assumption of binary sexual identities – men and women – with corresponding gender identities – male and female – is inadequate for a prevention response to HIV, so is the assumption that sexual minorities are all the same, and can be easily pigeon-holed. Policy makers need to know enough, and be sensitive enough, to reach all members of the population at risk from HIV.

Historical movements

The way that cultures have tried to make sense of people who do not fit the usual categories of female and male, has varied. A Thai origin story describes three sexes, the third sex/gender being *kathoey*, who is a distinct type of human being (Vitit 2005). In contrast, the response of Western societies has tended to ignore reality, classifying people into neat binary categories, and to persecute those who deviate from this scheme.

In the West, over the past three decades, gay liberation movements have forced mainstream society to recognise the existence of homosexuality, and the rights of people who have same-sex sexual relationships. Similarly, 'second wave' feminism[5] forced society to recognise differences in the roles and status of women and men, and to respond to the rights claims of women. Both these movements emphasised a common experience of marginalisation, in order to make the case for equality and liberation.

The analysis and strategies of second wave Western feminists generated a huge critique by women around the world, whose sense of themselves was not explained only in terms of their relationships to men. Instead, women in developing countries asserted their identity as complex individuals with multiple identities including, but not reducible to, gender identity. They rejected the 'women in development' (WID) approaches of the 1970s for their failure to understand or address this reality.

The crude binary distinctions between men and women, male and female, and heterosexuality and homosexuality were challenged by Judith Butler, who in her (1990) book *Gender Trouble* shows how attributing any single 'identity' to a human being is inevitably constraining and limiting, and is a way of policing people's behaviour. Judith Butler's work demonstrates the great disservice that second wave feminism did to women who did not identify as heterosexual. They had been subsumed under the category 'women', which made their specific issues invisible and unworthy of consideration and redress.

The political implications for other sub-groups whose difference is ignored or denied are obvious. Identity labels do have certain pitfalls, in that there is always variation that they miss; however, they have emerged as politically salient. The two main gender-variant groups studied in Phnom Penh are 'short hair' men who have sex with men, and 'long hair' *Srei Sros*. Both groups strive, albeit in different ways, for the right to live their identities. Within these identities, collective concepts of rights may emerge. Their struggle is to reduce their marginality and replace it with freedom. Coming out and naming themselves is a claim to power.

The role of development and community organisations

It is widely agreed that the HIV/AIDS pandemic has generated a new urgency about understanding people's sense of themselves as sexual beings, and some of the most high-profile debates on the issue of sexual identities have occurred in the context of HIV (Jagose 1996). AIDS may in fact be leading to new understandings not only of identity, but also of politics, community, and agency (Edelman in Jagose 1996).

Borthwick (1999) researched differences between Western and Asian styles of HIV-related development work. In one case she studied, Thai *kathoey*, referred to as 'gay men', worked with villagers to organise care for AIDS patients. Identity politics with a sexual-rights platform as put forth in the West would be foreign to this group. In another case, Borthwick (1999) noted that the project *Chai Chuay Chai* (men helping men), a Western-funded project in northern Thailand, introduced a completely new model of making change. The project used peer educators to provide safe-sex education and condoms to men frequenting gay bars or cruising areas. The project aimed to stimulate the formation of a gay community (Western style), another completely new development (Borthwick 1999).

NGOs working in Phnom Penh, with a Western focus on building communities and collective agency (the ability to effect changes and achieve rights through group activities), are currently facilitating the 'emergence' of people with different sexual and gender identities. Though the impetus towards fostering ideas of community rights and citizenship did not arise from within the local groups, and the movement incorporates foreign terms and ideas, the effects seem to be working for these groups. Discussion has been stimulated, and marginal people have been exposed to new concepts of rights and claims to membership in civil society. These outcomes are positive aspects of globalisation.

A sense of emerging power coming from a group with a shared identity is most evident among the 'short hairs'. The MHC project and drop-in centre legitimate their existence and condone their going out publicly as men who have sex with men, a new and heady experience. Their non-confrontational approach has been politically successful beyond what they could have imagined a few years ago. When, in the course of outreach work, fieldworkers were threatened by violence from 'real men', MHC met with the respective commune chiefs and received complete co-operation and security support (interview, 30 September 2004). Likewise, they now enjoy a good relationship with the police stationed at Wat Botom Park (observed 30 September 2004). Informants marvelled at how much progress has been made over the last three years in ensuring that men who have sex with men are able to be visible, and protected by the authorities.

Although it is still impossible for sexual minorities to have successful long-term relationships due to discrimination, it is getting better for them. A good relationship between men is one in which they can discuss their feelings, help each other, and provide mutual support so that 'their mind is OK' (Mao Kimrun, 28 May 2005). Recently (former) King Norodom Sihanouk spoke out on behalf of sexual minorities and as a result, it is now legally possible for two men (sic) to marry (Pak Kim San, Khmer Development Freedom Organization, 9 August 2004; interview, MHC, 1 October 2004). This development is quite unusual for the region, and encourages the larger society to be more tolerant, allowing sexual diversities more freedom. It may herald a new era for the coming generation, in which they may be able to form partnerships of their own choice.

Srei Sros have a more difficult life than 'short hairs' because they blatantly transgress conventional definitions of man and woman. Friendships provide support, but they do not yet have an identity-based project or drop-in centre from which to build a community. Though they are at the very margins of society, their strength is that they have always existed in Cambodia. Thus, culturally, they have a right to exist. In this modern age of HIV and violence, however, simply living is a radical act.

The two groups are located differently, and may continue to define themselves in opposition to each other. However, it is not too difficult to envision a coalition developing as the discourse matures. Coming out of the shadows presents new challenges and hurdles as well as new potentials for happiness. After rights have been won and the context thereby changed, identities will be free to shift/morph/multiply, and together form a new context.

Conclusion

An approach to HIV/AIDS prevention that ignores gender diversities is faulty from a public-health point of view, and unjust from a human-rights point of view. It is a form of gender bias deriving from a way of understanding human beings that excludes and marginalises those who differ from the norm. Small efforts by NGOs do not fill the gaps that governments are expected to fill. But questions arise: should the Ministry of Women's Affairs include *Srei Sros* among its constituents? Would inclusion dilute gender-equality claims of the masses of women who struggle with conventional problems? Would it cause more backlash against the very notion of gender equality? The debate about whether *Srei Sros* are women or men is likely to continue as long as gender is conceived within the terms 'female' and male'. But as the debate proceeds, recognition of gender diversities by the authorities, and corresponding gender-sensitive HIV efforts, must be furthered on the dual grounds of public health and human rights.

Because of the threat that HIV/AIDS poses to everyone in Cambodia, it creates a totally new context in which to recognise and accept sexual diversities. Except for *Srei Sros* who have always existed openly, non-normative people have, until now, had little reason or motivation to identify themselves. But, there is no question that they are there, in all their dizzying diversity.

A concern with labels and identities is a very new development; a direct result of discussions about sexualities in relation to HIV. It is important that policy makers as well as practitioners stretch their gender concepts and become familiar with local gender realities.

This article was originally published in Gender & Development, *volume 14, number 2, July 2006.*

References

Altman, D. (1995) 'Political sexualities: meanings and identities in the time of AIDS', in R. G. Parker and J. H. Gagnon (eds.) *Conceiving Sexuality: Approaches to Sex Research in a Postmodern World*, New York: Routledge.

Borthwick, P. (1999) 'HIV/AIDS projects with and for gay men in northern Thailand', in P. A. Jackson and G. Sullivan (eds.) *Lady Boys, Tom Boys, Rent Boys: Male and Female Homosexualities in Contemporary Thailand*, Chiang Mai, Thailand: Haworth Press and Silkworm Books.

Brummelhuis, H. T. (1999) 'Transformations of transgender: the case of the Thai kathoey', in P. A. Jackson and G. Sullivan (eds.) *Lady Boys, Tom Boys, Rent Boys: Male and Female Homosexualities in Contemporary Thailand*, Chiang Mai, Thailand: Haworth Press and Silkworm Books.

Butler, J. (1990) *Gender Trouble: Feminism and the Subversion of Identity*, London and New York: Routledge.

Catalla, T. A. P., Sovanara Kha, and G. van Mourik (2003) *Out of the Shadows, Male to Male Sexual Behaviour in Cambodia*, Phnom Penh: KHANA.

De Lind van Wijngaarden, J. W. (1999) 'Between money, morality and masculinity: the dynamics of bar-based male sex work in Chaing Mai, northern Thailand', in P. A. Jackson and G. Sullivan (eds.) *Lady Boys, Tom Boys, Rent Boys: Male and Female Homosexualities in Contemporary Thailand*, Chiang Mai, Thailand: Haworth Press and Silkworm Books.

Earth, B. with Chea Fung (2005) *Gender and HIV/AIDS in Phnom Penh, Cambodia: Situation Analysis and Action Plan*, Occasional Paper No. 64, Pathumthani, Thailand: Urban Management Programme for Asia and the Pacific.

Gender, Education and Advocacy, Inc. (2001) 'Guide to Using the Gender Variance Model', www.gender.org/resources/dge/gea02007.pdf (last accessed August 2007).

Girault, P., T. Saidel, Song Ngak, J.W. De Lind van Wijngaarden, G. Dallabetta, F. Stuer, S. Mills, Or Vathanak, P. Grosjean, P. Glaziou, and E. Pisani (2002) *Sexual Behavior, STIs and HIV among Men Who Have Sex with Men in Phnom Penh*, Cambodia 2000, Phnom Penh: FHI.

ISNA (n.d.) 'How Common is Intersex?', Intersex Society of North America, www.isna. org/faq/frequency (last accessed August 2007).

Jackson, P. A. and G. Sullivan (1999) 'A panoply of roles, sexual and gender diversity in contemporary Thailand: an introduction', in P. A. Jackson and G. Sullivan (eds.) *Lady Boys, Tom Boys, Rent Boys: Male and Female Homosexualities in Contemporary Thailand*, Chiang Mai, Thailand: Haworth Press and Silkworm Books.

Jagose, A. (1996) *Queer Theory: An Introduction*, New York: New York University Press.

The Kinsey Institute (n.d.) The Kinsey Institute for Research in Sex, Gender, and Reproduction, www.kinseyinstitute.org/about/ (last accessed August 2007).

Koyama, E. (2003) 'Guide to Intersex & Trans Terminologies', Survivor Project, www. survivorproject.org/basic.html (last accessed August 2007).

Mann, J. and D. Tarantola (1998) 'Responding to HIV/AIDS: a historical perspective', *Health and Human Rights* 2(4): 5–9.

MWVA (2003) *Policy on Women, the Girl Child and STI/HIV/AIDS in Cambodia*, July, Phnom Penh: Ministry of Women's and Veterans' Affairs.

NAA (2001) *National Strategic Plan for a Comprehensive and Multi-Sectoral Response to HIV/AIDS 2001–2005*, Phnom Penh: National Aids Authority.

Pilcher, J. and I. Whelehan (2004) *Fifty Key Concepts in Gender Studies*, London: Sage.

Tarr, C. M. (1996) *People in Cambodia Don't Talk about Sex, They Simply Do It! A Study of the Social and Contextual Factors Affecting Risk-Related Sexual Behaviour among Young Cambodians*, prepared for UNAIDS, Phnom Penh: Cambodian AIDS Social Research Project.

Vitit (2005) 'LGBT: Towards Equality in Thailand', Opening Speech of the Thai LGBT Community at a conference on Sexualities, Genders and Rights in Asia organised by the Office of Human Rights Studies and Social Development at Mahidol University and the Asia Pacific Queer Network, Bangkok, Thailand, 7–9 July 2005.

Wichayanee Ocha (2006) 'Gender, Sexualities and Identities in the Global–Thai Sex Sector: Focus on Male and Male to Female Transgender Sex Workers', unpublished doctoral dissertation proposal, Klong Luang: Gender and Development Studies, Asian Institute of Technology.

Notes

1 A cruising place is where people go to look for sexual contacts. In Phnom Penh, they are largely city parks, the Mekong riverside, or certain bars. Cruising places may attract the full range of genders and sexualities, because people are looking for different things.

2 The Western tendency is to see sex as either male or female; gender as either masculine or feminine; and sexuality as either heterosexual or homosexual. The binary distinction between heterosexuality and homosexuality was debunked by Alfred Kinsey, whose research in the 1940s and 1950s found a continuum of sexual orientation among American men and women (The Kinsey Institute, n.d.). Kinsey's findings opened up new possibilities of ways to understand gender, sex, and sexual identity, but still saw sexuality as located along a continuum between binary opposites. Asian concepts, in contrast, seem less constrained by binary constructs.

3 Transgender is an umbrella term used to describe *visibly* gender-variant people who have gender identities, gender expressions, or gendered behaviours not traditionally associated with their given sex at birth (Gender, Education and Advocacy, Inc. 2001). 'MtF' (male-to-female) and 'FtM' (female-to-male) are two of the common ways trans people describe themselves. 'Trans' can be used as an umbrella term (Koyama 2003).

4 At this time, there is only one Cambodian *Srei Sros* who has had sex-change surgery. She is a famous and rich film star named 'Puppy'.

5 Second wave feminism was a period of feminist collective political activism that emerged in the late 1960s and early 1970s and focused on the liberation of women from patriarchally defined society. The 'second wave' is contrasted with the 'first wave', which dated roughly from the mid-nineteenth century to the 1920s and focused on women's enfranchisement through the vote (Pilcher and Whelehan 2004, 144).

7 Young men and HIV

Doortje Braeken, Raoul Fransen, and Tim Shand

Introduction

The face of HIV is increasingly young. Currently, more than 33 million people are living with HIV worldwide (UNAIDS 2007) and almost a quarter of this group are under the age of 25 (UNAIDS 2004a). Young people (aged 15–24) now account for 50 per cent of new HIV infections (WHO 2006). Although young men account for a significant number of those living with HIV, the international response to date has placed greater emphasis on the vulnerability of young women and girls. While this approach remains necessary, particularly in areas such as sub-Saharan Africa where more than 75 per cent of those living with HIV are female, it also risks excluding the very group whose involvement is essential if we are to be successful in turning the tide on HIV; namely, young men, particularly those living with HIV (UNAIDS 2004b).

The importance of directly engaging young men and boys in shaping the response to HIV and AIDS is clearly reflected in the 1994 International Conference on Population and Development (ICPD) Programme of Action. Paragraph 4.27 highlights the link between human sexuality and gender relations. It states the need for special efforts to be made to emphasise men's shared responsibility for, and promote their active involvement in: responsible parenthood; sexual and reproductive behaviour; family planning; prenatal, maternal, and child health; and the prevention of sexually transmitted diseases, including HIV. Commitments to make such efforts have been reiterated in several international declarations such as the Political Declaration of the 23rd session of the UN General Assembly in 2000 (Beijing + 5) and the Declaration of Commitment on HIV/AIDS, adopted at the 26th Special Session of the General Assembly on HIV/AIDS (June 2001).

Such engagement is seen as essential to upholding the reproductive rights of young women and helping to protect them (and their children) from HIV, given the unequal balance of social and economic power between young men and women in many parts of the world which, for instance, often makes it difficult for women to negotiate the use of a condom with a male partner. But this engagement is also essential to improve young men's own health outcomes. The social construction of masculinity in many parts of the world leads young men to take risks with their sexual health: men are expected to be sexually active from an early age; they often view condom use as inhibiting sexual fulfilment; and they are more likely to have multiple partners simultaneously, because sex is seen as a male 'necessity' and 'uncontrollable'. The pressure that young men face from men and women in society to conform to these patterns of behaviour, and the risky behaviour that such attitudes support, make encouraging young men to find alternative, safer ways of expressing their sexuality even more important.

In addition, the growing number of young men living with HIV requires us to seek new ways of specifically supporting this group, and to better understand their behaviours, addressing their needs and enabling them to continue living positively, loving, and working as agents of change in the midst of an increasingly complex epidemic.

This chapter seeks to present a brief overview of the issues relating to HIV and the lives of young men, here defined as those between the ages of ten and 24. It considers why young men's involvement in the prevention of HIV is important, how their sexuality and socialisation impacts on such involvement, and why we haven't previously effectively reached young men. It will also discuss issues regarding improving information and services, and give some examples of how existing programmes address the needs of young men. The discussion also gives special attention to the realities of young HIV-positive men and concludes by providing key recommendations for engaging with young men to ensure safe sexual health and well-being for all.

Why focus specifically on young men and their needs?

It is now recognised that it is important to work specifically with young men while they are in the process of forming their own views about their roles and values in relation to sexual behaviour and sexual health, in order to instil in them positive notions about sex, sexual relationships, equality, and the roles and responsibilities of men and women. As the ICPD Programme of Action highlights, at this early stage, young men can be more effectively influenced to understand and follow safer sexual practices, such as delaying sexual initiation, reducing the number of sexual partners, and engaging in alternative non-penetrative sexual activity. They can also be encouraged to obtain accurate information on HIV, sexually transmitted infections (STIs), and other sexual-health issues, discuss their feelings and concerns, and seek confidential advice, ideally establishing the habit of utilising sexual and reproductive health (SRH) services throughout their lives.

Working with men and boys from an early age also helps to improve and increase the use of contraception. The unequal balance of social power between young men and women in many parts of the world often makes it hard for young women to negotiate contraceptive use with their male partners, and leaves young men as key decision-makers in this regard. If good contraceptive practices are instilled in men during their youth and adolescence, this would undoubtedly have very positive immediate and future outcomes for both men and women. For example, adolescent males in the USA who used condoms during their first sexual encounters were more likely to become consistent users of condoms thereafter (Sonenstein *et al.* 1995, referenced in Barker 2000). In other words, sex education needs to start early in order to prepare boys to be healthy, supportive partners in mutually respectful relationships.

There is now a greater understanding than there used to be of the fact that male gender norms and values influence both sexual decision-making and health-seeking behaviours among young men, which in turn affect the health and well-being of their sexual partners, be they girls, young women, or other young men.[1] Despite this, many HIV interventions to date have lacked a focus on the influence that gender roles and gender inequities have on sexual decision-making. In addition, while there has been increasing research on gender-related risks and vulnerabilities to HIV, the majority of this work has focused on the specific needs and risks of young and adult women, and it is only in recent years that there has been greater analysis of the role of men, particularly young men, in HIV-prevention efforts (Nzioka 2001; Harrison *et al.* 2005). Further study in this regard is therefore required (Wood and Jewkes 1997).

Young men living with HIV also have their own specific SRH needs and desires. With an increasing number of young men testing positive for HIV, greater focus is needed on the specific prevention, treatment, and care required by this group, including psychosocial support on healthy living. This is essential given that young men can experience denial and isolation when they become HIV-positive, and thus fail to take the necessary precautions to prevent disease progression and protect others.

Clearly, therefore, working with young men on the full continuum of HIV services has direct benefits for the health of other men, women, and children. In working with young men it is nevertheless important to recognise that they are a diverse group at different stages of development, and with differing circumstances, needs, and problems. Such differing and changing needs for information and services should be appropriately reflected within the work of service providers and policy makers.

Why we haven't been reaching young men

Earlier discussions on the need to work with young men and boys often centred on how 'male involvement' could improve women's reproductive health. Although important, particularly as it relates to encouraging men and boys to assume full responsibility for their sexual health and behaviour, this perspective implied the passive involvement of young men. This failed to recognise the need for a proactive attempt to understand young men's motivations for, and benefits from, engaging in efforts to promote greater gender equity and the health of others. What is more, within this 'male involvement' framework, men have often been perceived as the key 'problem' in relation to the spread of HIV and other STIs, again impeding efforts to engage them as constructive partners. Traditional sex education and HIV prevention and information programmes, for example, often focus (intentionally or otherwise) on young women, and do not adequately address the needs of young men, such as concerns they might have about masturbation, penis size, maintaining erections, and premature ejaculation – all key reasons young men cite for not wanting to use a condom (Family Health International 1998).

Because of this focus on women's reproductive health, SRH clinics are often perceived, and indeed sometimes promote themselves, as 'feminine spaces', where staff and service users are overwhelmingly female. This often means young men feel uncomfortable visiting SRH clinics, which in any case frequently lack services catering for their specific needs. In addition, few clinics have staff who are appropriately trained and have the capacity to offer the necessary counselling and advice; in particular, there is a shortage of male service providers, with whom young men may feel more comfortable talking, and who thus have a vital role in helping young men articulate their thoughts and feelings about sex and STIs. Where such services exist they are often provided on a short-term basis, and are not integrated into the core activities of SRH programmes.

A good example of a successful SRH programme targeting young men comes from the Swedish Family Planning Association (RFSU). Within the existing SRH clinic, a special time slot is allocated for young men to visit. Experience there shows that unless they think they have an STI, young men do not really feel that they have to go to a doctor, but they are willing to have a physical examination if they are assured that the purpose is to confirm that 'everything is ok'. This type of knowledge could help inform future successful programmes; in addition, involving young men themselves in the design of SRH programmes would be another way of addressing some of these challenges.

Young men, masculinity, and HIV

It is important when discussing young men's SRH, particularly in the context of HIV, to acknowledge the different forces and influences that shape masculinities. For instance, in many cultures, the 'stereotypical male' is expected to possess characteristics of strength and bravado, pursue adventure, and be secure in his knowledge and feelings of sexuality in order to be a 'real man'. Although these processes affect young men in different ways – creating varying levels of needs, wants, and vulnerabilities – it is essential to find ways to support all young men to feel positive about themselves and to accept their place in society. This self-acceptance is essential to enable young men to respect others and develop a sense of responsibility for shared experiences with (young) women and other (young) men. The realities of a young man's world, however, include anxieties and secret concerns about social failure, his body, and his sexuality. The struggle between these hidden anxieties and the fear of not conforming to socially defined constructs of masculinity often leads to patterns of behaviour which have a negative impact on young men's SRH, as well as placing young women at increased risk of HIV infection (Barker 2000; Rivers and Aggleton 1998). In their desire to prove that they are 'real men', boys and young men may view girls and women as sex objects, condoning coercion, violence, and abuse to obtain sex, and equating sexual prowess and multiple sexual partners with manhood. This means that, as studies across different cultures have shown, men tend to have more sexual partners than women and thus on average experience more exposure to risk situations and can be expected to infect more partners in a lifetime (UNAIDS 2000). In some societies in Africa for example, men have an average five-year period between their sexual debut and marriage. During this period, young men are likely to have more sexual partners than young women, who are more likely to marry when they are young, and to marry older men. This greater number of partners, combined with inconsistent condom use, means that both men and their female partners are vulnerable (Barker and Ricardo 2005). In contrast, equally rigid views about acceptable feminine behaviour mean that women are expected to be passive and innocent on matters related to sex and are thus placed at heightened risk of HIV infection (Rivers and Aggleton 1998).

Gender role socialisation has thus perpetuated HIV infection risks for both young men and women, while significantly shaping the expansion of the epidemic (*ibid.*). For example, research in Brazil, applying the 'Gender Equitable Men Scale', which measures men's attitudes towards women's rights, the role of men as fathers, sex, violence, and homosexuality,[2] found that men who held more traditional beliefs about gender and the roles of men were more likely to have used violence against women and to report having had an STI (Pulerwitz *et al.* 2004). In this context, there is a clear need for more research on young men's attitudes to gender and sexuality, to understand how these shape sexual behaviour, and attitudes to women. These topics have been substantially ignored, particularly on qualitative levels, and it is only more recently that a growing literature concerned with male sexuality has begun to emerge.

One example of a programme that has sought to integrate analysis of gender, and how it is understood in everyday life, into HIV prevention is the 'Living for Tomorrow' project, implemented in Estonia. This project explored the dilemmas and challenges in implementing gender-focused HIV-prevention education in contexts where people have barely begun to explore critically the realities and consequences of the gender system they lived in during the Soviet period. It also looked at the difficulties in encouraging adult facilitators to become 'youth-focused' and use participatory education methods. Results from the project included a leaflet on 'How to Bridge the Gap Between Us? Gender and Sexual Safety', written and illustrated by the young people themselves, as well as a manual that offers some simple learning activities that can help HIV educators or trainers develop young people's critical gender awareness, a crucial element for effectively promoting safer sexual behaviour (Lewis 2002).

Adolescence is also a time when homophobic attitudes and behaviours can form, often deriving from efforts to exaggerate masculinity and reject traits that are perceived to be feminine. These attitudes have led to human-rights abuses and violence frequently perpetrated by young men. At the same time, however, the formative years of adolescence are the time when young men may be most willing and receptive to developing more equitable concepts of masculinity and more informed and sensitive attitudes and perspectives regarding their roles and responsibilities in SRH and intimate relationships. Indeed, these changes are already happening, and need to be further supported and normalised. For instance, in Nicaragua, the Association of Men Against Violence (AMAV) works with men on issues around masculinities and attitudes to gender roles, making the link between these and acceptance of violence against women. Part of this includes encouraging young men to confront their own homophobia, and to analyse how this shapes their view of 'acceptable' masculine behaviour (CIIR 2002).

Moving forward: young men and HIV prevention

The growing recognition that preventing HIV and AIDS is not possible without reaching men and boys has led to increasing programmatic efforts, interventions, and research around the world seeking to engage this group in questioning social and cultural norms, addressing gender inequalities, and promoting better health outcomes and rights for themselves, other men and boys, women, and children. This section presents a number of examples of such interventions in the areas of safer sex, condom use, young gay men, the SRH needs of young men living with HIV, fatherhood/care-giving, and young men as agents of change.

Safer sex

Even when young men (and young women) possess adequate information about safe sex, they still engage in risky behaviour. Research has shown that while factual knowledge of HIV transmission is important, it is not a sufficient predictor of safe sexual behaviour (Moore and Rosenthal 1993). Working to fill this gap between knowledge and behaviour thus requires an understanding of what actually leads adolescents to engage in unsafe behaviours.

The Horizons programme 'Reducing Young Men's HIV Risk and Violence Against Women by Promoting Gender-equitable Norms and Behavior' in India has been developed by CORO for Literacy, an India-based NGO, and Promundo, a Brazilian NGO. The programme conducted research to examine the impact on young men of promoting gender equity as part of an HIV-prevention programme. The research began with a qualitative investigation into how young men construct their gender identities. The questions included how masculinity is understood and expressed by young men in India and how gender-equitable norms and behaviours, including those related to violence and HIV and STI risk reduction, could be promoted among young men.

When asked about masculinity, the young men participating in the formative research described the physical and social attributes of a 'real man'. Overall, a 'real man' was characterised as someone who is handsome, strong, muscular, and virile. Sexual potency was seen as an important way for men to establish superiority and control over women. The young men often referred to women as 'items' or 'objects', as if they belonged to men. To demonstrate sexual power, men commonly reported using coercive behaviour, including touching, making derogatory comments, whistling, and harassing women in public places. It was evident from the research findings that condom use did not figure prominently in the lifestyles of the young men. Sex often happened in a hurry, and there was little thought given to using a condom.

This information guided the development of a group-based intervention that was piloted in three large slum communities in Mumbai. Using exercises and materials that were adapted from Promundo's Program H in Brazil (Barker and Nascimento 2002), the India programme aimed to change negative aspects of masculinity and reduce risky sexual behaviour among young men. Men who participated in the programme were found to be less supportive of negative gender stereotypes, reported less sexual harassment, and were less prone to risky behaviour. Based on this pilot programme, the scheme has been expanded to target over 1,000 young men in urban Mumbai and rural settings in the state of Uttar Pradesh. In some areas, group education activities are combined with a community-based and gender-focused 'lifestyle' social-marketing campaign to reinforce gender-equitable safe sex and HIV-prevention messages. The campaign promotes a gender-sensitive and violence-free lifestyle for young men in the community, and consists of street plays, posters, pamphlets, banners, and a service and information booth (Verma *et al.* 2006).

Condoms

The male condom has always been presented as simple to use, but this may not reflect what young men actually feel. Research in Denmark and the Netherlands shows that fear of premature ejaculation or a loss of erection could be a factor in discouraging the use of condoms among young men (Vennix *et al.* 1993). For many young men the condom may often also be presented in a way that exacerbates their own fears and confusion, making them reluctant to experiment with using one. Using wooden models of penises in sex-education classes, for instance, may cause young men to perceive that an erection should always be like foolproof machinery, i.e. rock hard all the time. While the information given with the female condom includes details on what to do when things go wrong or when you have a problem, such 'trouble-shooting' information is not provided with male condoms. It is essential that such issues are addressed if we are to increase access to, and utilisation of, male condoms.

Condoms can also be made more accessible if they are designed and marketed in a way that is culturally appropriate. In Australia, koori[3] were closely involved in the brand development of Snake Condoms, which were then launched in 2004 during National Youth Week at a free music event. While this brand was specifically targeted at young indigenous Australians aged 16–30, the young people involved in the project had a strong desire to produce a brand that would appeal to all young people, as they viewed STIs, HIV, and unplanned teenage pregnancy as issues impacting the broader community, regardless of skin colour or cultural background.[4]

That said, appropriate branding and information leaflets can only ever have a limited impact: the condom will only work as a prevention tool for HIV infection where it is part of a comprehensive package of other tools and information, available to people where and when they need it, and adjusted to their realities. This includes information on when it is safe not to use a condom (for instance, those in longer-term relationships may no longer want to use condoms because they feel 'safe', or want to have different kinds of sexual experiences), what a positive or negative HIV test result means for safe-sex decisions, and the impact of anti-retroviral treatment on the risk of transmission.

Young gay men

'Am I gay?' is a question young people in the Western world have more freedom to ask, now that there is much more openness and honesty about discussing lesbianism and male homosexuality. There is a growing feeling among many younger people of both genders that sex is there to be enjoyed in various forms, and that they do not really want to be categorised as being heterosexual, bisexual, lesbian, or gay.

However, there are still large numbers of young men (and women) living in countries where there is a stigma attached to being homosexual. Questions about sexual orientation are seen as offensive and a challenge to a young man's masculinity, making it extremely difficult for young men to answer honestly, or even to admit their true sexuality to themselves. The stigma and discrimination faced by men who have sex with other men plays a significant role in increasing men's vulnerability to HIV, as it not only limits access to appropriate information but also access to SRH services.

In HIV-prevention activities, the term 'men who have sex with men' (MSM) is used to describe men who identify themselves as heterosexual and have sex with other men. However, in many contexts, this term is inappropriate, and does not reflect the complexity of sexual relations between men, or the role of gender and other power dynamics in shaping those relations. For instance, the NAZ foundation in India expresses their concern with the use of this term in South Asia, where many instances of men having sex with men are shaped by gender, sex, and/or age roles. The penetrating partner often sees himself as a 'man', while the penetrated partner tends to be perceived, and perceives himself as not a 'man'. Thus in both cases, the term 'men who have sex with men' is not really appropriate (Khan 2004).

There is much that can be done both to improve access to information and services for men who have sex with men, and to encourage changes in attitudes towards homosexuality. In Western countries, a considerable amount of effective HIV-prevention work has been carried out with gay men since the advent of HIV and AIDS in the early 1980s. Much of the work has involved groups and communities of gay men themselves. Many men have felt motivated to get involved because they have seen their friends and partners become infected with HIV. Others have felt that their particular needs have been ignored by mainstream health education and promotion.

A good example of a particularly effective intervention is the Mpowerment project, which was implemented in California, USA. This project was based in a gay community and involved young gay men working in gay venues and other community settings, to initiate discussion groups and informal conversations with their peers to promote safer sex. Young gay men were involved in the management, design, and implementation of the project, which helped ensure its relevance to other young gay men. The project successfully raised awareness about the risks of unprotected anal sex throughout the community, and reduced unprotected anal sex among young gay men (Kegeles *et al.* 1996). Similarly, in the UK the 'Committed to youth' project, health-promotion services, and the commercial sector came together to distribute safer-sex information and condoms through special events in night clubs.[5]

Different types of intervention have been used with young gay men who do not use gay social and community venues and groups, and who do not, or cannot, identify themselves as gay at all. For example, in Belgium a Flemish HIV-prevention organisation has developed a project which involves young gay men who have just 'come out' in working with other young men who are unsure, or exploring their sexuality. In this project the young gay men are trained and equipped to run 'house parties' and other small events in community venues and people's homes, where young men can come together to talk about their feelings and experiences. Safer-sex materials and condoms are made available (Forrest and Reid 2001).

The sexual and reproductive health needs of young men living with HIV

With one in every two HIV infections occurring among young people, it is necessary to examine critically what this means for our prevention efforts, and also to look beyond young people as a mere target group for such prevention efforts. Young men living with HIV are to be considered a resource in understanding what drives risky behaviour, and involving them in programming may lead to tools and interventions which are better tailored to the realities of these individuals, as well as helping to prevent future infections.

Programmes often do not recognise the complexity of an individual's sexuality. HIV makes this sexuality even more complex. It does not, however, make a young person any less of a sexual being. Young men (and women) living with HIV have the same sexual desires and rights to a full and satisfying sex life as anyone else, but they also require specific services and support. As such, a number of programmes are increasingly adopting a 'positive prevention' approach.[6] This includes a set of actions which help people living with HIV to protect their sexual health, and live longer and healthier lives; look after their partners; avoid other STIs; delay HIV or AIDS disease progression; avoid transmitting HIV to others including their children; and reduce stigma and discrimination. To better address the needs of young men living with HIV, existing services and prevention approaches should be re-orientated, and the needs and rights of people living with HIV placed at the centre.

When it comes to starting new relationships, young seropositive[7] people are not only struggling with the issue of HIV status disclosure, but also debating whether or not to initiate relationships with people who have not been diagnosed with HIV, and to understand what sexuality actually means, and how they perceive themselves as sexual beings. Just like anyone else, a young man living with HIV wants his partner to understand who he really is. He also wants to be perceived as a person beyond his HIV status. Some seropositive people choose to look for partners and relationships with other HIV-positive individuals. Others, for a variety of reasons, do not limit themselves to seropositive potential partners.

People living with HIV who choose to engage in relationships with other HIV-positive people (seroconcordant)[8] do so for a variety of reasons. Many choose seropositive partners because there is an *understanding* of what living with HIV entails on a day-to-day basis. They believe that in a seroconcordant relationship, their partners can relate to how they feel and what they may be going through physically, mentally, and emotionally. There may also be less of a fear that they will be rejected on the basis of their HIV status. Dating and communication may be easier with other HIV-positive people because disclosure is usually not an issue.

Young Positives is an international network of young people living with HIV. Regardless of the great disparity between the global North and the global South, Young Positives' experience is that the issues HIV-positive young people face are similar, wherever they live. Young Positives supports young people living with HIV in concrete ways, for instance through establishing support groups. It also advocates for their rights and needs, pressing for youth-friendly support and services that reflect the realities of young people's lives, and the meaningful involvement of young people at all levels of decision-making. Through these activities, valuable experiences and lessons learned are gathered that can inform programming at all levels of the prevention and care continuum. The utilisation of such resources is essential to work on addressing the needs of young men living with HIV.

In Romania, a support group for young people born with HIV, established with support from Young Positives, rapidly evolved into an organisation advocating the rights of young people living with HIV. Their focus is on fighting stigma in medical and social settings, HIV in the workplace, and raising awareness among the general public by working with the media. However, despite being involved in national government HIV-prevention campaigns and having support from national networks of people living with HIV, UN country offices, and international partners, the group has found it difficult to develop an agenda around sexuality. One reason for this is that other partners involved do not recognise the importance of providing support in this area.

The Young Positives network in Mexico also changed in a short period of less than a year from providing peer support to acting as a powerful advocate on the issues faced by young people living with HIV. This came to a sudden halt when the leader and founder of the organisation was murdered in early 2005, for being open and outspoken about being gay and HIV-positive. This has had a tremendous impact on subsequent efforts to mobilise young gays and young people living with HIV in Mexico, as it proves that involvement in such mobilisation can unfortunately have terrible consequences.

Fatherhood and care-giving

Young fathers, in general, have an essential role to play both in the physical and psychosocial development of their children and in the prevention of HIV and AIDS. In order to highlight the specific role, and needs, of fathers living with HIV, the International Planned Parenthood Federation (IPPF), together with the Global Network of People living with HIV (GNP+), developed a publication entitled 'Fulfilling Fatherhood: Experiences from HIV Positive Fathers'. This publication provides real-life stories from around the world on the ways in which HIV-positive fathers are acting as key agents of change in the HIV epidemic, and in addressing stigma and discrimination. It also highlights the additional needs among HIV-positive fathers for information and support in child-birth, disclosure, and remaining a role model for their children.

Young men also have an important role to play in caring for those both infected, and directly affected, by HIV and AIDS. Through training and supporting young volunteers, organisations such as the Movement of Men Against AIDS in Kenya (MMAAK) are creating a new cadre of male home-based carers, and breaking the stigma regarding the role of men in HIV care and support.

Young men as change agents

Young men, particularly those living with HIV, are not only clients with their own health needs or partners with joint responsibility for the health and well-being of their children and families, but also agents of change in promoting gender equality in health. Given that men are often the gatekeepers to the effective implementation and scaling-up of policies, programmes, and services, young men play an essential role as advocates and role models in undertaking interventions to empower men and boys (and women) to better understand, support, and address HIV and AIDS within their communities.

The Young Men as Equal Partners (YMEP) project is being implemented by RSFU and IPPF in Tanzania, Uganda, Kenya, and Zambia. It seeks to build the skills of young male peer educators to enable them to undertake outreach work and encourage men in the community – particularly community and religious leaders and others in senior positions – to act against HIV and AIDS. This programme is leading not only to health improvements at a local level, such as a reduction in reported STIs and school pregnancies and an increase in condom use, but also to the development of a national policy environment more conducive to the involvement of men in preventing HIV.[9]

Some conclusions and recommendations

It is clear that we need to work with young men, particularly those living with HIV, to address their needs, instil in them notions of gender equity, and prepare boys to be healthy, supportive partners in mutually respectful relationships. This will arguably bring very positive immediate and future outcomes for both men and women.

Better addressing the needs of young men requires that we broaden and rethink our existing package of services to specifically cater for their sexual health and HIV-prevention concerns, including sexual dysfunction, infertility, and STI treatment. We must ensure that we are innovative – seeking to reach young men at the most appropriate times and in the most convenient locations – and that our approaches are comprehensive, and based on a thorough understanding of the local and specific SRH needs of men and boys. Such provision will require training for counsellors and service providers on addressing these needs.

Young men living with HIV have the same sexual health needs as anyone else, and therefore require equal access to existing services and support. But they also have more specific needs because of their HIV status. These include:

- more information about treatment, as well as psychosocial/positive living support for young men living with HIV (particularly immediately after a young man tests positive);

- greater focus on prevention services for young men living with HIV, and services to address their specific SRH needs, including information regarding serodiscordant relationships;

- family planning, including how young men living with HIV can support the process of preventing parent-to-child transmission of HIV;

- specifically tailored information and support for key populations (of young men and women) most vulnerable to HIV – sex workers, men who have sex with men, and intravenous drug users living with HIV.

In addition, an important focus needs to be on empowering young gay and bisexual men, and men who do not identify as gay but who have sex with other men, and on providing safe legal and social environments.

Young men also have key roles to play as role models, advocates, and peer educators in speaking out to others, particularly males, about HIV prevention and treatment, and should be provided with support to fulfil these roles. The meaningful involvement of young men living with HIV is essential, both to ensure that we have a more effective impact, and as a way of reducing HIV-related stigma and discrimination.

We need to start early. The process of sexual socialisation begins during infancy, and the messages on gender roles inform and shape attitudes and behaviour within a socially defined framework of boundaries and opportunities. Interventions with young men must also not be short-term, but ongoing and integrated processes built within approaches which identify and address the needs of men at every stage of their lives.

Young men are not a homogeneous group. Recognising their diversity in terms of their socio-economic circumstances and their sexual identity and lifestyle are crucial to ensuring that SRH rights initiatives respond to the real needs of young men. This must include responding to the specific needs of young male fathers, and recognising that this contact acts as an 'entry point' to addressing other HIV and SRH issues with this group.

Specific strategies are required to encourage greater use of condoms among young men, and ensure that such interventions are located within a broader focus on men's sexual health. Positive and realistic messages which look beyond the risks and promote the freedom to love safely are essential when educating boys about condom use. These messages must also place the sexual realities and desires of young men at the centre, and address the specific concerns among this group that may undermine or discourage effective and consistent condom use.

Young men do not live in a vacuum, but within community and cultural contexts where very specific understandings of acceptable gender roles and behaviour operate. Thus, young men cannot and should not be targeted as an isolated group. Working with young men does not, therefore, mean isolating women, particularly young women and girls. Interventions and efforts to increase safer sex and voluntary counselling and testing (VCT) service utilisation among young men, and to better address their sexual health needs, should not be at the cost of essential services for women (young and older). In addition, involving young women is essential to increasing their support for work with young men, and will provide them with the opportunity to explore the ways in which they may reinforce traditional 'masculinities', as well as develop their understanding of the wider social benefits of addressing male SRH.

Building on existing lessons learned to seek to strengthen the evidence base for this work is essential, not only to ensure more effective programming but to enable this work to influence at a policy level. Lessons from these interventions, research, personal experiences, and the differing settings and types of HIV epidemics, must be shared widely. This will help to support the sustainability of interventions and lead to the development of models – based on approaches which have been shown to work and display positive attitudinal and health outcomes – which can be replicated in different contexts.

Finally, meaningful partnership with young men in SRH initiatives as decision-makers, programme partners, and evaluators is vital for responding to their needs, ensuring that they are no longer isolated from the SRH rights arena. To have any meaningful and long-term impact, we need to understand and acknowledge fully the crucial importance of supporting young men (and young women) in making safe and healthy decisions, and develop programmes in partnership with them, based on their true realities.

References

Amaro, H. (1995) 'Love, sex, and power: considering women's realities in HIV prevention', *American Psychologist* 50(6): 437–47.

Barker, G. (2000) 'What about boys? A literature review on the health and development of adolescent boys', Geneva: WHO, www.who.int/child-adolescent-health/New_Publications/ADH/WHO_FCH_CAH_00.7_en.pdf (last accessed November 2007).

Barker, G. and M. Nascimento (2002) 'Project H: working with young men', Poster Exhibition: The XIV International AIDS Conference: Abstract No. MoPeD3609, www.iasociety.org/Abstracts/A3807.aspx (last accessed November 2007).

Barker, G. and C. Ricardo (2005) 'Young men and the construction of masculinity in sub-Saharan Africa: implications for HIV/AIDS, conflict, and violence', Social Development Papers: Conflict and Reconstruction No. 26, Washington DC: The World Bank, www.promundo.org.br/Pesquisa/Young%20Men%20SubSaharan_Web.pdf (last accessed November 2007).

Campbell, C. A. (1995), 'Male gender roles and sexuality: implications for women's AIDS risk and prevention', *Social Science and Medicine* 41(2): 197–210.

CIIR (2002) 'Men changing: power, masculinities and non-violence from Latin America to Europe', London: CIIR (now Progressio), www.aidsportal.org/repos/Men%20Changing-%20Progressio.pdf (last accessed November 2007).

Cohen, S.L. and M. Burger (2000) 'Partnering: a new approach to sexual and reproductive health'; Technical Paper No. 3, New York: UNFPA, www.unfpa.org/upload/lib_pub_file/170_filename_partnering.pdf (last accessed November 2007).

Family Health International (1998) 'Reaching young men with reproductive health programmes', *In Focus*, December, www.fhi.org/en/Youth/YouthNet/Publications/FOCUS/InFOCUS/youngmen.htm (last accessed November 2007).

Forrest, S. and D. Reid (eds.) (2001) 'HIV/AIDS prevention for young people: models of good practice from the European Member States', Utrecht: European Information Centre AIDS & youth NIGZ.

Harrison, A., J. Cleland, E. Gouws, and J. Frolich (2005) 'Early sexual debut among young men in rural South Africa: heightened vulnerability to sexual risk?', *Sexually Transmitted Infections* 81: 259–61.

Kegeles, S.M., R.B. Hays, and T.J. Coates (1996) 'The Mpowerment Project: a community-level HIV prevention intervention for young gay men', *American Journal of Public Health* 86(8): 1129–36.

Khan, S. (2004) 'Masculinities, (homo)sexualities, and vulnerabilities in South Asia', Lucknow: Naz Foundation International, www.nfi.net/NFI%20 Publications/ Essays/2006/masculinitiessouthasia.pdf (last accessed November 2007).

Lewis, J. (2002) 'Learning to relearn givens: exploring gender strategies in Estonia', in A. Cornwall and A. Welbourn (eds.) *Realizing Rights: Transforming Approaches to Sexual and Reproductive Well-being*, London: Zed Books.

Moore, S. and D. Rosenthal (1993) *Sexuality in Adolescence*, London and New York: Routledge.

Nzioka, C. (2001) 'Perspectives of adolescent boys on the risks of unwanted pregnancy and sexually transmitted infections: Kenya', *Reproductive Health Matters* 9(17): 108–17.

Pulerwitz, J., G. Barker, and M. Segundo (2004) 'Promoting healthy relationships and HIV/STI prevention for young men: positive findings from an intervention study in Brazil,' Horizons Research Update, Washington DC: Population Council, www.popcouncil.org/pdfs/horizons/ brgndrnrmsru.pdf (last accessed November 2007).

Rivers, K. and P. Aggleton (1998) 'Adolescent Sexuality, Gender and the HIV Epidemic', New York: UNDP HIV and Development Programme, www.undp.org/hiv/publications/gender/adolesce.htm (last accessed November 2007).

Sonenstein, F., J.H. Pleck, and L. Ku (1995) 'Why young men don't use condoms. Factors related to the consistency of utilization', Washington DC: The Urban Institute Washington.

UNAIDS (2000) 'Men and AIDS, A Gendered Approach: 2000 World AIDS Day Campaign', Geneva: UNAIDS, http://data.unaids.org/pub/Report/ 2000/20000622_wac_men_en.pdf (last accessed November 2007).

UNAIDS (2004a) 'At the Crossroads: accelerating youth access to HIV/AIDS interventions', Geneva: UNAIDS Inter-agency Task Team on Youth and Young People.

UNAIDS (2004b) '2004 Report on the Global AIDS Epidemic', Geneva: UNAIDS, Executive Summary available at http://data.unaids.org/ Global-Reports/Bangkok-2004/UNAIDS_Bangkok_press/GAR2004_pdf/ GAR2004_ExecSumm_en.pdf (last accessed November 2007).

UNAIDS (2007) '2007 AIDS Epidemic Update', Geneva: UNAIDS/WHO, http://data.unaids.org/pub/EPISlides/2007/2007_epiupdate_en.pdf (last accessed December 2007).

Vennix, P., P. Curfs, and E. Ketting (1993) *Condoomschroom: jongens over seksualiteit, anticonceptie en SOA-preventie*, NISSO studies, nr. 14, Delft: Eburon.

Verma, R.K., J. Pulerwitz, V. Mahendra, S. Khandekar, G. Barker, P. Fulpagare, and S.K. Singh (2006) 'Shifting support for inequitable gender norms among young Indian men to reduce HIV risk and partner violence', Horizons Research Summary, New Delhi: Population Council.

WHO (2006) 'Preventing HIV/AIDS in young people: a systematic review of the evidence from developing countries', Geneva: UNAIDS Inter-agency Task Team on Youth and Young People, www.who.int/child-adolescent-health/New_Publications/ADH/TRS/ISBN_92_4_120938_0.pdf (last accessed November 2007).

Wood, K. and R. Jewkes (1997) 'Violence, rape and sexual coercion: everyday love in a South African township', *Gender & Development* 5(2): 41–6.

Notes

1 For a fuller discussion of this, please see: Amaro (1995), Campbell (1995), Cohen and Burger (2000), and Pulerwitz *et al.* (2004).

2 The Gender Equitable Men Scale (GEM) is a psychometric evaluation of a 24-item scale to measure attitudes toward gender norms among young men. Indicators on gender norms are related to sexual and reproductive health, sexual relations, violence, domestic work, and homophobia. Higher GEM Scale scores are significantly associated with contraceptive use and lower levels of self-reported partner violence.

3 'Koori' or 'koorie' is the term used by some indigenous Australians in the south-eastern part of Australia to describe themselves.

4 Marie Stopes Australia: www.mariestopes.org.au/country-aust-proj2.html (last accessed November 2007).

5 Avert: www.avert.org/aidsyounggaymen.htm (last accessed November 2007).

6 Positive prevention is defined as prevention for, and with, people living with HIV.

7 Seropositive is used here to describe someone who has tested positive for HIV, and seronegative is used to describe someone who has tested negative for HIV.

8 A serocondordant relationship is a relationship between two individuals of the same HIV status (i.e. both negative or both positive; www.thebody.com/content/art14009.html, (last accessed December 2007).

9 For information on this programme, see www.rfsu.se/programmes(1).asp (last accessed November 2007).

8 HIV-positive African women surviving in London: report of a qualitative study[1]

Lesley Doyal and Jane Anderson

In sub-Saharan Africa, around 60 per cent of people infected with HIV are female (UNAIDS and WHO 2004). In other parts of the world, women from African countries also carry a heavy burden of HIV infection. In the UK, for instance, around 75 per cent of all women diagnosed as HIV-positive in 2003 came from Africa (UK Health Protection Agency, Centre for Infection 2004). Yet we know very little about these women's circumstances, or their needs. This article reports on a study exploring the daily lives of HIV-positive African women receiving medical care in London. It examines the complex choices they face in living with the disease, and the constraints that limit their options. It describes the strategies they adopt for their own – and their families' – survival, in difficult circumstances so far from home.

The research method involved the recruitment of a sample of HIV-positive black women from different African countries, from outpatient clinics at four east London hospitals. All the women were aged 18 and over, had been diagnosed as HIV-positive for at least six months, had attended the clinic in the period January 2000–June 2001, and had lived in the UK for at least six months. Approximately 80 per cent of women who were approached were willing to be part of the study. They completed a semi-structured interview, lasting between one and three hours. Most reported experiencing the interview as a valuable opportunity to talk about their own situation, and to be listened to. All expressed their willingness to be contacted again should the study be taken further.

Findings from the survey: an overview

Sixty-two women from 11 different countries took part in the study. Their age ranged from 20 to 58 years old. The average age was 33. They were a well-educated group compared with the UK population as a whole, with 12 per cent having finished primary school, and 61 per cent having completed secondary education. Twenty per cent were university educated, and seven per cent had postgraduate qualifications. Only 12 of the 62 women were working. Four were students, and 46 were unemployed.

When asked why they had come to the UK, some women stressed the new opportunities they expected to find in London. A number talked about poverty at home, while others mentioned the pursuit of business plans. Only three identified the need for medical care as a reason for coming to the UK. A number of women, from countries in east and central Africa in particular, mentioned political pressures at home. Many of these feared for their safety because of their own actions, while the remainder felt they were in jeopardy because of the political activities of other family members, usually husbands or fathers.

About a third of the women were asylum seekers at the time of interview. Sixteen of them had either compassionate or exceptional leave to remain for between one and five years, 12 had been granted indefinite leave to remain, and a further six had British nationality. Two described themselves as illegal immigrants, and one as a visitor. Most of the women (73 per cent) had been in the UK for more than a year. Seventeen had been in the UK for less than 12 months, and it was these women who were most likely to be asylum seekers at that time.

A Burundian woman involved in the research related her reasons for being in the UK as follows: 'When I first came, I came seeking asylum. I had problems in my country. There was fighting and this guerrilla thing and ethnic tribes fighting each other, which I didn't know. I didn't know that my husband was involved somehow, somewhere, in those groups. So we were attacked and they tied him up and took him, so I ran for my life' (W2, Burundi).

Twenty-eight of the women were in a relationship with a male partner. Of these, 11 were cohabiting. The vast majority of the women (55) were mothers, but only 39 of them had children living with them. Others had left their children in Africa in a variety of circumstances, and some were unaware of what had become of them. Around half of the women had HIV-negative children, 12 had at least one positive child, and in 13 cases the HIV status of the children was unknown.

A majority of the women had already experienced at least one profoundly traumatic life event. These included rape, murder of partners and family members, and various other forms of persecution. One woman from Zimbabwe said: 'I was raped – that's how I contracted it. When I was so young there was this political issue, that's when I was abused. I was detained for 30 days and every day raped by different men – I felt I was robbed of my life' (W62, Zimbabwe).

Twenty-seven of the women spoke of direct experience of HIV-related death and ill health in close relatives or friends, and eight had experienced the death of at least one child from HIV. A Malawian respondent told us: 'When my son died my whole world like turned into dust before me, I was like, this is the end of me. It was like there is nothing' (W12, Malawi).

Listening to the stories of these women, it was clear that many different factors were shaping their lives. First and foremost, their potential fertility meant that they had to face a range of difficult decisions about sexuality, pregnancy, and child-bearing. At the same time, their options were also constrained by their own and other people's expectations of how they should behave as female partners, wives, and mothers. These women were also migrants, living with the challenges posed by life in a strange country. Finally, they were HIV-positive, with all of the social and biological implications that come with such a diagnosis.

Being a woman with HIV

For most African women, motherhood is a major source of identity and legitimacy. Many pointed out that failure to have children can have profound economic and social consequences, including divorce or desertion. A Zambian woman told us: 'If you have no children, it means you are less of a woman' (W47, Zambia).

But there was also a reluctance, among the women we spoke to, to bring a child who might be HIV-positive into the world. For some, this was compounded by anxiety that unsafe sex might put the potential father at risk, as well as the fear that pregnancy might exacerbate their own disease. A Tanzanian woman said: 'For me who's not got a child...I love kids, and I can't wait to have a child...Then I could pass it on to that child...and you can't give your child breast milk you know, we are women. I want to explain all these things as a woman you know, and you can't. It's very difficult' (W18, Tanzania).

Mothers are traditionally seen as the moral guardians of society. This meant that many of these HIV-positive women were afraid of being stigmatised for not living up to social expectations. This was reflected in the ways in which they told their stories:

'When I gave out my blood I was very sure I was negative, because I was healthy and strong. But when I got the results I was shocked, I was shocked. I had to do another test, at least two tests to be sure that it's true that I'm HIV-positive.'

W9, Kenya

'You ask yourself, where did I go wrong? I was just a perfect, perfect lady. You know there are some ladies who go into the pub, they expose themselves to find men, but I wasn't the type of lady. I was the type of a lady who was so reserved. But well, there it is.'

W57, Zimbabwe

Most of the women had become mothers before their diagnosis, and 39 had their children living with them. Their experiences of mothering with HIV were complex and contradictory. Many were raising their children in considerable economic poverty, without the support of an extended family, and often as single parents. A Ugandan respondent commented: 'I just have to stand up for my kids so I'm the mum, I'm the dad, I'm the auntie, I'm everything...So they need me' (W28, Uganda). For many, these responsibilities were made even more difficult by continuing concern about their children's health. Another Ugandan woman told us: 'I had thought he was going to be born dead so I was delighted when he was alive, but when I was told he was positive, my world shattered' (W21, Uganda).

Guilt was often especially debilitating among those who were compelled to leave children behind in Africa. Many women were trying to support their children by sending money home from their own limited resources. But most found their (unavoidable) failure to fulfil what they and others saw as their maternal role deeply distressing: 'I wanted to bring my children over because that is the thing that is really eating me up, it's still eating me up you see, because I am here and my children are on their own – they don't even have a father because he died a long time ago, and they are living on their own' (W50, Zambia).

For these women, the reality of motherhood brought both intense pleasure and inevitable pain. The experience of parenting brought many burdens. But at the same time it gave many a reason to live and to survive the disease. The Tanzanian woman quoted earlier stated: 'I am going to live for the sake of my baby. That's it' (W18, Tanzania).

Migrant status and HIV

The women in the study were all living far from their countries of birth. Though many were financially better off in the UK than they would have been at home, they still had limited access to a range of economic, social, and cultural resources compared with many of those they saw around them. In addition, many had severe problems with their legal status as immigrants to the UK. This affected their capacity to make realistic choices about both the present and the future. A Ugandan respondent talked of the paralysing effect of her fear and insecurity arising from unresolved immigration issues: 'Every ring of the doorbell, they've come to deport me, that's what it feels like, the sight of a police car, are they looking for me, you know; that's the kind of life you have to live and definitely with the virus you don't need that' (W38, Uganda).

Whatever their financial circumstances, all the women in this study were constrained by the fact that the UK was not their home. But for those living on state benefits, economic problems were paramount, with the support for asylum seekers especially low. Not surprisingly, many of the women talked about the difficulties they faced in making ends meet, especially when their illness generated special needs.

A Kenyan respondent said: 'A Freedom Pass is from 9 o'clock and maybe you want to go to hospital and you have an appointment at 9 o'clock which means you have to start travelling early, travelling and you don't have money to pay for it' (W9, Kenya). Another respondent, also from Kenya, commented that: 'It is really horrible because you want to go and buy your African food from the African shop, but you can't buy with the food vouchers...You have to go to the supermarket' (B13, Kenya).[2]

Housing conditions, too, were frequently inadequate. Prior to resolution of their immigration status, many of the women had lived in multiple occupancy properties often with small children. Their anxieties were often compounded by the constant fear of deportation. Our respondent W9, quoted in the last paragraph, told of her experience: 'It was difficult because of the nine-year-old...[we shared]...a single room...and then having to share a bath and toilet with strangers, and we shared with one person who was a drug user, every time you get in the bathroom there was syringes everywhere'.

Living with the effects of HIV

The third element shaping the lives of these women was the HIV infection itself. Not surprisingly, many reported that it led to feelings of depression and anxiety. These women have a potentially fatal disease, and many have seen relatives and friends die from it. Their access to drugs was experienced as highly uncertain, and therefore they felt that their very survival was threatened. One Ugandan woman described the state of 'just not knowing, you know, I mean, yes we're all going to die but just not knowing, you know, what will start it off, when it's cold you dress really, really warm...I'm just so scared of picking up anything that I will not go to a hospital, I just want to sort of stay clear of anything' (W23, Uganda).

Many women reported that they usually felt physically well. But about a third described physical symptoms, which limited their everyday life. They reported tiredness, side effects of medications, and unpredictable periods of illness and disability including deteriorating sight, and mobility problems. A number commented on the distress they felt when HIV affected their capacity to work. For example:

> 'I want to try and do whatever I can to get my life back. I want to put my knowledge, the things I've studied and my skills into practice. I don't want to just sit there and be on benefits, I want to be useful.'
>
> W50, Zambia

> 'It's so difficult because I would like to go back to work but all days are not the same, sometimes you can work, you can't work,...I would like to be working, because as well I need my freedom and I want to work freely.'
>
> W10, Kenya

Many of the women reported that their sense of themselves was radically changed by the reality of their illness. Not surprisingly, the experience was often a negative one, with the diagnosis seeming like an immediate death sentence:

'I've seen so many people at home die of HIV. I have on my mother's side about five people died of HIV and I saw them wasting away, so it's like death.'

W24, Uganda

'It's really changed my life. I don't know how to say it, it's amazing, there's never a day that I don't cry, you know.'

W3, Cameroon

'It's more than a shock to know you have HIV. You feel that life has come to an end, and yet you are still breathing.'

W3, Cameroon

But the shock of diagnosis could have good as well as bad consequences. For many, the diagnosis led them to re-evaluate their lives. They thought hard about their priorities, and about how best to use the time and energies remaining to them. A respondent from Zimbabwe told us: 'What I used to take for granted I don't take for granted anymore. If I'm doing something I always think oh maybe this is the last time I will be doing this. Let me do it properly' (W61, Zimbabwe).

Managing life with HIV

A major issue for all infected with HIV is to decide who should know. All the women in the study were concerned about how to control information about their HIV status. They needed some people to know, but not others, and were always scared of the response. Ten of the women had told no one at all outside the health-care team about their diagnosis. Some women indicated that they had received more support than they had expected when disclosing their status. However, most were afraid that they would be stigmatised.

Drawing on their experiences – both 'at home', and in African communities in the UK – the women talked about the extreme hostility often occasioned by a diagnosis:

'Even now, it is very hard to tell somebody I am sick, because like our community they take it as a curse, or like you misbehaved or went out with somebody, like they take you as a prostitute, it is an attitude which is very bad that we have.'

W47, Zambia

'Mostly, people say that it's witchcraft, that's what they believe.'

W7, Kenya

About a third of the women reported direct experience of HIV-related stigmatisation, including rejection by husbands or partners, eviction from their home, and denial of contact with children. When this was combined with the hostility many experienced as African migrants in the host community, the impact on mental health was often profound:

'I don't think you can ever come to terms with it, with HIV. Because in yourself you can come to terms with it but society doesn't allow you to, it's like society is fighting you all the time from all kinds of directions.'

W34, Uganda

'You see, if you tell your brother he will want to tell his wife, he tells his wife, his wife is going to tell her sister, the wife tells her sister, the sister wants to tell her friend. Before you know it, the whole community has talked of it.'

W15, Nigeria

Six women reported that they had made a conscious choice not to disclose their status to past or present sexual partners. The main reason given was the need to protect themselves from being abandoned or from physical or verbal abuse. A Kenyan respondent said: 'It took me about 11 months to tell him. I had prepared myself in case he throws me out of the house' (W9, Kenya).

Most women faced particular problems in deciding what to tell their families. Telling parents was seen as especially difficult, since most were back home in Africa. Imparting the news on the phone was often said to be impossible, yet travel constraints meant they were unable to do it face to face. Another Kenyan respondent said: 'If today I tell my mum I'm HIV-positive, within one week my mum would die' (W8, Kenya). A Zimbabwean woman said: 'If my passport comes back, I think I will go back home for a holiday, then come back, maybe that's when I will tell him and my mum' (W55, Zimbabwe).

Disclosure to children was always a matter of great concern, and most tried to avoid it as long as possible: 'I told my mum and she said for God's sake spare that boy, he's a very sensitive boy, so I would advise you not to tell this boy at the moment, let him grow up, and then he grows up and you are still alive, then maybe one day you sit him down and tell him' (W31, Uganda).

Relative success in establishing and maintaining a social life was linked to views about disclosure of HIV status. Some women managed to sustain very full social lives despite the diagnosis, and friends were very important to them. But they also talked about the need to compartmentalise friendships between those who were positive and those who were not: 'My life has changed since I found out I was HIV-positive – I have very few friends now and the friends I have are also HIV-positive...I don't feel comfortable sitting in the company of somebody who doesn't understand what I'm going through and hiding medication because you don't know who is coming to your house and what that person is going to think of you' (W9, Kenya).

But for the many who felt that they could only protect themselves and their family if they kept their HIV status secret, it was hard to sustain close relationships that were based in part on a lie. Hence, they preferred to retain a degree of separateness. Two typical views were: 'I have to keep a distance because I have to watch what I say, sometimes I might say something which would push my friend out, away, so I have to like be very careful' (W27, Uganda), and: 'I do have friends, but at the end of the day you have to cope and struggle on your own' (W19, Uganda).

Many of the women said that the lack of a male partner was one of the most difficult things they had to face. They wanted to be in an intimate relationship, but perceived the obstacles to be very great. For many, the lack of friends and of a partner resulted in physical and emotional isolation that was very difficult to bear. A Ugandan respondent expressed this dilemma of needing intimacy yet not feeling able to confide totally as follows: 'If I have to be in an affair, a relationship, I don't want a positive person, I want a person who's well, but the disclosure, to tell somebody that, I don't want to be heartbroken, I've been heartbroken, so my fear is to fall in love again' (W30, Uganda). A Nigerian woman stated: 'I can't bear this cross all alone. I need to share it with somebody...Most of the time you are the only one that knows your problem, and that drives you crazy at times' (W15, Nigeria).

Using health services

The women in this study described the health care in specialist London units as a major resource in their survival strategy. Many contrasted the right to treatment in the UK with the lack of care in their own country:

> 'They give you all the support when something is going wrong, they tell you something is wrong, they don't like just write your notes and chuck you the medicine. No, they will explain to you.'

W35, Uganda

> 'They [HIV clinic staff] are very kind. They have feelings towards us, very kind people...You know you mix with them and they have a chat and joke around, and that makes you feel at home.'

W31, Uganda

Some did find the clinic environment depressing, saying that frequent visits reminded them of their diagnosis. Several reported that doctors tried to explain aspects of care that they did not want to hear, and some were afraid of being recognised by others. However, most rated the HIV services they received very highly, and many travelled long distances to stick with familiar clinical teams.

Two-thirds of the women interviewed had experience of taking anti-retroviral (ARV) drug therapy. A number pointed out that their living conditions sometimes made compliance with drug regimes difficult. But despite their difficulties, most of the women remained extremely committed to taking these drugs. A Ugandan respondent told us: 'It was horrible...I got side effects, diarrhoea and vomiting...so I had to be really strong, you know, really, really persevere...I was just so determined I wasn't going to change...I knew my body would adjust. I just had this strong feeling that it would adjust and it did' (W23, Uganda). A Kenyan woman stated: 'I had to go on medication immediately, and it was very hard because you are living with somebody whom you haven't told and to have to take this medication, either with meals or after meals, and some have to be kept in the fridge, so I felt no, it was too much for me. But I managed to do it' (W9, Kenya).

These women had access to drugs that they would be very unlikely to obtain in their home countries. But unless they gave up the treatment, most would be unable to return to the families they had left behind. Hence the medication enabled them to survive, but often as reluctant migrants, and not necessarily in circumstances of their own choosing. A Zambian woman told us: 'I've been like cut off you know...It would have been really nice for me to go back and get back my job, go back to my family, go back to my friends...my home, the sunshine' (W50, Zambia).

Looking towards the future

Some of the women were understandably depressed, and found it hard to envision the future. Many were especially affected by their inability to return home without risking their lives. However, the most common theme to emerge was the desire to do something active, which would allow them greater control over their own lives. Despite the huge difficulties they faced, many of the women showed great determination and considerable optimism about new treatment possibilities. They were still looking towards the future and showed considerable resilience in trying to shape the best possible options for themselves and their families:

'I'm not gonna let this wear me down, I'm not gonna let it kill my spirit, or stop me from doing what I have to do, I just have to move on, you know.'
W39, Nigeria

'I don't think of death, I'm planning, I'm planning to study to get my degree, I'm planning to start to get a job.'
W30, Uganda

'I'm looking to the rest of my life, I don't know where, where is the end of my life or what, I don't know, but I just say, when I wake up in the morning I say, oh yes, thank you Lord, I'm here.'
W60, Zimbabwe

This article was originally published in Gender & Development, *volume 14, number 1, March 2006.*

References

UK Health Protection Agency, Centre for Infection (2004) *Survey of Prevalent HIV Infections Diagnosed (SOPHID) 2003*, London.

UNAIDS and WHO (2004) *AIDS Epidemic Update 2004: December 2004*, Geneva.

Notes

1 This chapter is a shortened and amended version of L. Doyal and J. Anderson (2003) *My Heart is Loaded: African Women with HIV Surviving in London*, available from the Terrence Higgins Trust (0845 1221 200) or downloadable from: www.tht.org.uk/informationresources/publications/policyreports/myheart584.pdf (last accessed August 2007). We would like to extend a particular thank you to all the women who gave their time to share complex and often painful life stories.

2 Asylum seekers in the UK are given their state benefits as vouchers rather than cash, and are only allowed to 'spend' them in certain shops.

Part III
Practical multiple approaches

9 Mitigating impacts of HIV/AIDS on rural livelihoods: NGO experiences in sub-Saharan Africa

Joanna White and John Morton

Introduction

In sub-Saharan Africa, around 26.6 million people are believed to be living with HIV/AIDS (UNAIDS/WHO 2003), while the estimated number of children orphaned in the region as a result of the epidemic stands at around 11 million (UNAIDS 2002). The aggregate impacts of AIDS are increasingly visible, and include dramatic reductions in life expectancy, the loss of adult workers in every sector, and a striking increase in the number of orphans and other vulnerable children (UNICEF 2002).

At household and community levels, the increasing ill-health and mortality of large numbers of 'prime-age' adults who had played a fundamental role in income generation, the protection of assets, and social reproduction, have severe repercussions. The composition of households is transformed and dependency ratios increase as adults grow sick and die, and as orphans are taken in to be cared for. This can place enormous pressure on resources. Furthermore, households are more likely to be headed by the elderly or by young people, many of whom are ill-equipped to cope (White and Robinson 2000). Over the long term, the transmission of knowledge concerning livelihood strategies and cultural and family heritage can be negatively affected.

A growing problem in many parts of Africa is the severe damage the epidemic is inflicting on rural communities. The direct loss of human capital and the diversion of resources and income to health-seeking and caring activities are having a critical impact on the various livelihood activities on which rural families depend for securing food and income, such as farming, fishing, food processing, petty trade, and the hiring out of labour.[1] Material and financial assets are gradually depleted due to decreasing incomes and the cost of health care, while traditional support mechanisms break down, heightening the vulnerability of rural communities to other shocks (De Waal 2002). This situation is exacerbated by the fact that many of those stricken with HIV/AIDS who were living in urban areas return to their native villages to be supported by relatives.

Given the current scale of the epidemic, the social and economic impacts of HIV/AIDS will persist long into the future, regardless of the success of HIV-prevention messages, increased access to anti-retroviral (ARV) drugs, or even the development of an HIV vaccine. Yet the lion's share of donor funding is still channelled towards preventive and curative health interventions. There have been few large-scale practical responses or shifts in policy aimed specifically at addressing the wider impacts of HIV/AIDS on livelihoods (Baylies 2002). The reasons for this are not clear. It is not simply a question of resources, although clearly the scale of the task and the probable associated costs may be daunting. There may be an assumption that generic development programmes and policies, which are aimed at mitigating poverty, can somehow address the impacts of HIV/AIDS (World Bank 1997); hence the continuation of existing approaches is understood to be a response in itself. Yet HIV/AIDS has served to expose the glaring inadequacies of standard development strategies to date, and their failure to ensure that the rights and livelihood needs of vulnerable population groups such as women, who are particularly affected by the epidemic, are met. Not only have clear links been established between patterns of HIV transmission and gender inequalities, but the impacts of the epidemic on families have also proved to be linked to prevailing discriminatory social and economic structures. For example, a large number of AIDS widows have been unable to uphold, or been actively deprived of, their rights over land. The limited access of women carers to credit and other resources has also posed significant constraints. Such realities suggest that existing development approaches may need to be re-examined in the light of the epidemic.

A crucial problem is that staff who are working outside the health sector are often uncertain about what should be done. Even individuals who have been allocated budgets explicitly aimed at tackling the impacts of HIV/AIDS on agriculture are often hesitant about how best to use such funding.[2] This raises the question as to whether current knowledge concerning effective means of addressing the social and economic impacts of HIV/AIDS is sufficient. At the same time, however, many local initiatives are now tackling the effects of the epidemic on rural communities. A key problem appears to be that information about such interventions is not widely disseminated. Personnel have limited time and resources to analyse and write up their work, so the lessons learned from project successes and failures are not shared, and experiences at grassroots level do not reach key decision makers.

This chapter details the main findings of a review to examine projects in sub-Saharan Africa dedicated to mitigating the impacts of HIV/AIDS on rural livelihoods. Carried out between 2001 and 2002 by the Natural

Resources Institute (NRI), the review aimed to raise awareness of approaches to counter the impacts of the HIV/AIDS epidemic in resource-poor settings. The chapter outlines the problems which current interventions are seeking to address, the focus of project activities, and perceived factors of success.

Projects reviewed

Field practitioners and other specialists recommended the projects to be reviewed and a total of nine projects were selected in four countries: the Kitovu Mobile Farm School Project, the UWESO Savings and Credit Scheme, the African Rural Development Initiative, the People with AIDS Development Association, and the National Community of Women Living with AIDS in Uganda; the Low External Inputs for Sustainable Agriculture (LEISA) and the ACORD Mwanza Urban Livelihoods programme in Tanzania; the Farmer Field Schools for Organic Cotton Production Project in Zimbabwe; and the Maluti Adventist Hospital HIV and AIDS Project in Lesotho. Project staff were asked to write up activities and experiences according to a checklist of questions, which resulted in a collection of case studies. Some of the details are summarised in Table 1.

Starting with people

NGOs, often local organisations operating on very small budgets, were found to be spearheading the response to the epidemic. The case studies revealed both how new projects had been developed in direct response to the impacts of HIV/AIDS, and also how existing work was adapted or new activities introduced as a result of growing awareness of the effects of the epidemic on intended beneficiaries. In every case, activities were planned with local communities through an often long process of stakeholder consultation. Despite the considerable time and resources devoted to this participatory process, it was found to be invaluable, providing project staff with the confidence that the activities promoted would best meet the needs of communities affected by HIV/AIDS. Moreover, in a number of cases the participatory planning process led to the identification of sectors of the population who are often unintentionally neglected by standard development programmes.

During the early stages of stakeholder consultation, communities were encouraged to highlight issues associated directly with HIV/AIDS which they felt to be of particular concern. The main issues identified are described below.

School dropouts

An increasing number of young people, especially orphans and teenage mothers, were being forced to leave school early due to pressures on family

Table 1: HIV/AIDS-related problems identified, target groups, and activities of projects reviewed

Organisation	Problem(s) identified	Target group(s)	Main activities
Kitovu Mobile Farm Schools, Uganda	High numbers of young people dropping out of school, especially orphans	Teenage school dropouts	Agricultural and vocational training Artisan apprentice-ship
Farmer Field Schools Project, Zimbabwe	Widows vulnerable due to limited labour and cash availability and lack of training in farm management	Marginalised farmers (principally widows and women heads of household)	Agricultural training and support Training on healthy living with HIV/AIDS
UWESO Savings and Credit Scheme (USCS), Uganda	High number of orphans. 'Care crisis' and limited resources for orphans and their carers	Orphans; guardians of orphans	Credit and loan schemes Vocational training
Low External Input for Sustainable Agriculture (LEISA) Project, Tanzania	Food insecurity Lack of income-gen-erating opportunities Pressure on resources due to PLWHA return-ing to rural home areas	Farmers Vulnerable groups, especially orphans and widows Local authority and organisational structures Fishing camp residents, and adolescents	Agricultural training in appropriate farming techniques Loans for purchase of locally fabricated transport technologies Loans for income-generating activities Awareness-raising on HIV/AIDS
African Rural Development Initiative (ARDI), Uganda	Teenage mothers dropping out of school and turning to sex work to raise income Vulnerability of PLWHA	Young mothers PLWHA Young people	Income support for young mothers Counselling and visits 'Life skills' education
Maluti HIV and AIDS Project, Lesotho	Psychological and social impacts of HIV/AIDS on PLWHA and their families	Sick people and orphans	Income-generating activities Home-based care Counselling Orphan care
People with AIDS Development Association (PADA), Uganda	PLWHA receiving little support	PLWHA	Home care and support Counselling Income-generating activities
National Community of Women Living with AIDS (NACWOLA), Pallisa Branch, Uganda	Vulnerability and stigmatisation of HIV-positive women Psychosocial problems faced by children of PLWHA	HIV-positive women Children of PLWHA Communities of PLWHA	Counselling, home care Support for income generation Memory project Awareness-raising

Organisation	Problem(s) identified	Target group(s)	Main activities
Mwanza Urban Livelihoods Project, Tanzania	Lack of credit for poor people Impact of HIV/AIDS on poverty	Poor and vulnerable households, including those headed by women and children; orphans; widows Groups at high risk of HIV infection PLWHA The wider community	Provision of micro-finance and business training Promotion of gender equity Environmental sanita-tion HIV prevention through Peer Health Educators

resources. As a result of their curtailed education, these young people were being left with limited means to support themselves, which increased the likelihood of their resorting to high-risk behaviour, such as transactional sex, to secure basic goods and cash.

Vulnerability of women

Women, often widows and elderly grandmothers, often bore the brunt of caring for people living with HIV and AIDS (PLWHA), while also being responsible for securing household food and income. Many of these individuals faced critical resource and information needs. For example, as a consequence of being widowed, women lacked the knowledge and resources needed to sustain the production of cash crops which had previously provided a vital source of income. In addition, their lack of access to credit, a long-standing constraint, had been exacerbated by the loss of male relatives who had had wider access to sources of financial support that had benefited the whole family.

Orphan 'care crisis'

While traditionally extended family and community support networks had absorbed orphans, the increasing number of children left without parents as a result of HIV/AIDS was placing such systems under considerable strain. Orphan-headed households were increasingly common and were at particular risk of abuse and destitution.

Vulnerability of PLWHA and their families

PLWHA and their families were not only experiencing the psychosocial impacts of chronic illness and bereavement but were also being stigmatised by the local community. This made these individuals less likely to seek support or to be open about their sero-status to their family and others. It also inhibited other members of the community from making use of HIV testing services.

Focus of activities

The interventions developed as a consequence of the stakeholder consultation process focused on four main areas: agricultural training; artisanal and vocational training; credit and loans provision; and HIV/AIDS awareness-raising, care, and support.

Agricultural training

Up to 80 per cent of people in the countries most affected by HIV/AIDS depend on agriculture for their subsistence (Villareal 2002). The epidemic is already having a serious impact on activities such as crop production and processing, and is thus undermining food and income security. Support to the agricultural sector is therefore crucial. Two principal (though not mutually exclusive) approaches to agricultural training and support were pursued by the projects reviewed. While these approaches may be appropriate for supporting poor farming communities in general, they can be seen to be responding directly to the particular impacts of HIV/AIDS.

Promotion of agricultural methods which use locally available materials and are adapted to farmers' existing resource base

The agricultural training undertaken focuses on promoting farming techniques which maximise production using materials that can be obtained locally at limited or no cost, minimise the intensity of labour and/or other input requirements, and lower the risks involved. This is in direct response to the fact that the human resource base and the resilience of capital and other assets have been depleted due to HIV/AIDS. Lowering, or smoothing, the levels of investment required while still sustaining productivity means that household food security is less at risk and incomes can be conserved. PLWHA and their families are therefore less vulnerable when household resources are diverted to pay for home care and medicines.

Clearly the techniques promoted to meet this end depend on the local context and agricultural system. Year-round agricultural production, for example, may be suitable only in some areas, but enables AIDS-affected households to spread the risks of their human and capital investments more effectively. The introduction of multiple farming systems enables farmers to cultivate their fields during the dry season, which can both enhance food security and income and reduce dependence on larger-scale inputs. This is in contrast with traditional, seasonal farming, which relies more on intensive inputs at specific times of the year.

Similarly, the promotion of strategies such as multi-cropping using carefully selected crops can reduce the need for weeding and other inputs. The use of locally fabricated transport facilities such as wooden wheel-barrows, and water conservation techniques can all save on household labour, which can then more readily be diverted to other activities, such as caring for the sick and earning income from alternative sources.

Encouraging crop diversification provides families with a wider range of goods for home consumption and sale. Training in horticultural production, for instance, provides farmers with the possibility of generating additional income on which they can fall back when other crops perform poorly.

A number of projects promote traditional food crops, which are nutritious and relatively cheap to produce. The production of such crops has declined significantly in many areas due to the push towards more market-oriented products. Traditional food crops can play a vital role in providing PLWHA and their families with a balanced, nutritious diet, and even prolonging life. Knowledge of the production and processing methods related to these crops often rests with the older generation, many of whom are responsible for caring for children orphaned as a result of HIV/AIDS. This indigenous knowledge is at risk of being lost to rural communities. In some cases, therefore, projects provide not only seeds and planting material but support the transmission of knowledge in order to stimulate a resurgence of such traditional crops.

Training for groups with limited knowledge and who have previously been excluded from such support

The demographic impacts of HIV/AIDS have led to a transformation in responsibilities. Orphans, teenagers, widows, and women more generally are now playing an increasingly critical role in heading households and securing livelihoods. Historically these social groups were excluded from agricultural support services, including government extension services. Also, young people, particularly orphans, are less likely to have benefited from hands-on training in agricultural methods from their parents and may not have considered farming to be a viable income-generating activity. By directing training towards these particular groups, projects can not only empower individuals and benefit families but also contribute to the local rural economy.

The Farmer Field Schools project in Zimbabwe, for instance, provides training to poor women farmers (many of them 'widows from AIDS' or nursing sick husbands or relatives) in the production of cotton, a cash crop for which men had traditionally been responsible. The field schools promote organic methods of cultivation which can reduce capital and, in some cases, labour requirements. The project has also taken active measures to revive the cultivation of traditional food crops. Home-garden production of millet, cowpea, bambaranuts, and pumpkin as well as the staple crop, maize, is supported through the provision of seeds, and education and training. The farmers' groups that have emerged as a result of this project have subsequently evolved into wider support groups that provide a forum for emotional support and the sharing of knowledge and labour.

The Kitovu Mobile Farm Schools Project in Uganda provides teenage school dropouts, including orphans, with new skills in sustainable agriculture, animal husbandry, and farm business. The project not only offers young women and men the opportunity to enhance the basic food security and income potential of their households, but also provides them with access to new, profitable agricultural techniques, thereby encouraging them to remain in rural areas and pursue farming as a viable livelihood option. The farm schools run for two years and involve intensive residential training and practical demonstrations using resources provided by local schools and communities. Groups of students are trained in a range of areas, including organic agriculture, small animal production, marketing, literacy, arithmetic, and record keeping. They put the skills they have learned into practice by farming on land provided by their families or guardians, or borrowing land from other community members. Box 1 offers a first-hand example of what the Kitovu Mobile Farm Schools Project seeks to achieve.

Box 1: Personal testimony from a graduate of a Kitovu Mobile Farm School

Both of N's parents died in 1990 when she was eight years old. She dropped out of school in 1998. In the same year she joined Kyanamukaaka Mobile Farm School as a trainee. She is now living with her elder sister. Before joining the Farm School, she was at home doing household chores. She had no source of income and there was little food at home.

'Due to lack of money I decided to become sexually involved with a senior secondary student from the next village to get money to help me meet some of the essential needs at home. When the Mobile Farm School was initiated in the area, I joined. I studied in the Farm School for two years (1998/2000) and graduated in December 2000 with a certificate and many skills acquired. In the Farm School I learned the basic facts about HIV/AIDS. From this knowledge, I came to realise that I was in danger of contracting HIV/AIDS and becoming pregnant if I carried on with my sexual encounters. With the knowledge acquired in modern agriculture and the information attained from the behaviour change programme in the Farm School, I have become self-reliant and I am able to meet the basic needs at home. I will not engage in casual sex again for money as I now know the dangers, and besides that, I have enough income from farming to support myself and the rest of the household. Nowadays other young girls and their guardians/parents come to me for advice and education.'

This project has made a significant difference to the food and income security of the households of the young men and women involved. At the time that the project was reviewed, at least 70 per cent of graduates were continuing to farm in their local areas and around 15 per cent of graduates had generated enough surplus income to purchase land. Some had even been able to fund their completion of formal education while still maintaining farming activities.

The relevance of the approach adopted by the farm schools project is evident from the fact that it has already been replicated by an NGO in Tanzania, although the curriculum has been shortened and adapted to a new context. The youth-based farmer groups that were initially established as a result of the Tanzania initiative have, with support from their local communities, begun lobbying village governments to recognise orphans' rights to land. This is an important development. The provision of agricultural training for groups made vulnerable by HIV/AIDS will have a sustainable impact only if there are parallel initiatives that ensure that such groups are provided with secure access to land.

Two other possible interventions in the field of agriculture which anecdotal evidence suggests are already occurring but which were not components of the particular projects reviewed are the design and construction of lighter and more manageable farming tools for women and children, and the provision of economic support for child-headed households to enable them to hire agricultural labour to carry out activities which are beyond their physical strength, such as land clearance. Other innovations are also likely to be taking place which have not yet been shared with the wider development community.

Artisanal and vocational training

As described above, it is increasingly common for children, particularly orphans, to be removed from school early due to lack of financial capital, and the need to care for sick family members and/or compensate for the loss of family labour. This leaves school dropouts with limited livelihood opportunities for their future. In response to this problem, a number of projects provide financial support and materials to enable orphans to train in fields such as teaching, nursing, carpentry and joinery, brick making and laying, commerce, and mechanics. One project in Uganda operates an apprentice scheme which provides funds to local artisans who then train orphans in carpentry, bicycle repairs, radio repairs, sewing, and mechanics; activities which enable beneficiaries to make a living in or close to their home community.

Other projects offer similar training and support but in the form of focused income-generation activities. The Maluti project in Lesotho, for example, trains groups in candle making to meet an identified market demand in South Africa; the project run by the National Community of

Women Living with AIDS in Uganda provides specialised training and support in small animal husbandry and marketing.

The potential problem of local skill saturation has not yet been an issue as most activities have been geared towards a consistent, identified demand. There is, however, a recognised need to ensure that projects innovate in terms of the activities they promote. Staff of one project, for example, observed that female orphans tend to be interested only in 'traditional' women's tasks, such as hairdressing and sewing, which are not always well-remunerated activities; nor do they always enable full economic independence. The NGO in question is now encouraging young women to diversify into new livelihood activities.

Credit and loans

Microfinance schemes aimed at enhancing the economic opportunities of vulnerable groups form an important component of a number of the projects reviewed. The credit provided has enabled beneficiaries to diversify into economic activities such as animal husbandry, horticultural production, and small business development. Even relatively small amounts of credit, such as the 30,000 Tanzanian shillings (around $17 at the time of the review) provided by one NGO to young mothers as part of a revolving fund, have offered new opportunities for clients. Most of the projects that operate loans disburse them to individuals through a system of self-selecting groups which share liability. This ensures local ownership over the intervention and instils peer pressure, which can discourage defaulting. In many cases such projects also provide training in functional literacy, book-keeping, and financial management, which has enhanced local capacity and self-esteem and enabled beneficiaries to build up relatively efficient and well-managed enterprises.

A number of projects direct their credit schemes towards women and/or guardians of orphans. For example, the UWESO Savings and Credit Scheme in Uganda is aimed at those who bear the brunt of the impact of HIV/AIDS. Women-headed households and orphans therefore comprise the majority of beneficiaries. The scheme works through self-selecting groups of five people who guarantee each other's loans. Ten groups make up a 'cluster', with both groups and clusters having elected leaders who hold specific responsibilities. Many clients use the credit provided to expand petty trade activities, often in relation to commodities in high demand such as maize, beans, fruit, general groceries, and charcoal. Other enterprises include hairdressing salons and drink stores. As income is consolidated, clients can use the funds to ensure that orphan dependants are able to stay in school and/or, in some cases, diversify into new business enterprises. By August 2001 over 12,000 households were benefiting from the initiative, which has empowered local communities not only by facilitating the generation of income but also through enhancing local leadership skills. In addition, a policy of 'breaking the silence' surrounding HIV/AIDS, which is promoted by UWESO staff in their discussions with clients, has resulted in less stigmatisation of PLWHA and their families.

There are clearly dangers in seeing credit alone as a 'quick-fix' solution to the problems posed by the epidemic (or, indeed, poverty itself). The experiences of the projects reviewed reveal how credit schemes need to be carefully designed in order for them to be responsive to the context of local livelihoods. For example, in the case of the UWESO project, loan defaulting in some regions resulted in the NGO creating new packages of smaller loans and offering more intensive training in business management for particular geographical areas.

The provision of microfinance to PLWHA and their families can pose further challenges. For example, there may be a high risk of default unless appropriate measures are in place. The provision of short-term, transferable loans (so relatives of PLWHA can take on credit responsibility if the original client dies), emergency funds to cover payments still outstanding when clients die, or insurance schemes, are some of the options pursued. There is a growing field of expertise in the area of microfinance for clients affected by HIV/AIDS (Donahue 1999; Donahue *et al.* 2001; Allen 2002) and the value of exploring alternative strategies, such as savings-led approaches, was recognised by project staff.

Some projects have faced a dilemma as to whether it is possible to introduce credit to the poorest and most vulnerable groups, such as seasonal migrants and transitory squatters, whose resource base is too limited or whose livelihood system too fluid to enable them to embark on sustainable new enterprises, even if they are given some seed money. In such circumstances it has been found that other support systems and interventions are required and social welfare is necessary to ensure that such groups do not fall further into poverty as a result of the impacts of HIV/AIDS.

Another approach is the direct provision of material assistance. In one of the projects in Uganda, for example, goats were provided to young mothers who had dropped out of school and were considered to be at risk of HIV infection because of their economic vulnerability. Goats are traditional assets in local communities and were intended to improve the food and economic security by providing the young women with a potential source of savings. However, an evaluation of this project found that many women sold their goats almost immediately for cash – their priority was clearly to gain immediate access to money to finance other activities. This experience highlights the need to address both immediate and long-term economic needs in AIDS-affected communities. Clearly in this particular case the development of a credit scheme for young mothers might have been more appropriate.

Awareness-raising, care, and support

All nine projects reviewed are responding to specific problems related to the impact of HIV/AIDS (or at least that the epidemic is known to have exacerbated). In addition, HIV awareness-raising activities and the promotion of discussions about the disease with target communities have also become an integral part of the work of some NGOs in order to counter stigmatisation and prevent the spread of the epidemic. A number of projects also undertake HIV/AIDS-specific activities, including counselling and the provision of support for PLWHA such as home visits, palliative care (massages etc.), as well as supplying food and blankets, and providing assistance with house building and home repairs. Such basic support can alleviate the various pressures faced by households affected by HIV/AIDS, and allow family members to pursue livelihood activities that can secure food and income more effectively.

The promotion of 'positive living' is also an important area. This includes education on healthy diets and the development of home gardens to enhance household nutrition. For PLWHA, information on the production and benefits of nutritious food to sustain their health offers hope, in contrast with the climate of fear often surrounding the epidemic.[3] 'Positive living' also involves supporting PLWHA in disclosing their sero-status to their immediate family members and friends and assisting them in organising their lives before they die by making a will, for example, and making plans for the future of their children. The creation of 'memory books' by PLWHA and their families is also a positive activity. It can assist young children in remembering their parents and their experiences together, raise their awareness concerning their ancestry, and ultimately enable them to cope more effectively with the bereavement they experience.

There is often a risk that the introduction of new support activities that are outside the initial brief of a project can become 'add-ons' of dubious quality, which divert scarce resources. Indeed, in the case of at least one of the NGOs consulted, staff concluded that it was more beneficial to communities to facilitate the introduction of HIV-prevention activities by another agency with particular expertise in this field than for staff to attempt to diversify into this area themselves. However, others found that the introduction of HIV awareness-raising, care, and support activities was enhanced by the relationships of trust already established with beneficiaries through earlier, practical areas of work. Existing livelihood interventions can therefore provide an effective entry point for other, more sensitive, areas of work.

Lessons learned

Staff involved in the projects under review highlighted a number of issues as having been especially important in contributing to the success of their work. These are outlined below.

Participatory, partnership-based approaches

A considered process of stakeholder consultation was a vital approach to devising new interventions. This process enabled the development of well-focused activities and the establishment of local commitment to new activities, all of which ensured projects had a greater chance of lasting impact. In addition, interventions were reviewed with beneficiaries on a regular basis and adapted according to changing needs. This responsiveness was considered a critical aspect of project success.

Countries whose national leaders have publicly acknowledged the problems posed by HIV/AIDS and the need for action have seen the benefits of this through changes in attitudes and behaviour (and, subsequently, HIV prevalence rates). Similarly, project experience revealed how involving influential community figures from the outset of project activities provided significant results. A reduction in the stigma faced by PLWHA was observed in projects where support from local political leadership was strong, for example. Furthermore, in Uganda, a decline in the cultural practices which are known to influence the spread of HIV, such as wife inheritance, were observed in some areas where traditional leaders had been involved in project development.

Project staff also found that working with adult 'gatekeepers' (those who provide information to and influence the decisions of young people), has been important. The involvement of adults who are trusted, admired, and chosen as intermediaries by young people has been an effective way of increasing inter-generation dialogue on HIV/AIDS. It has created a positive environment for young people at risk of HIV exposure to discuss the issues that affect them, and enabled orphans and other vulnerable children to share their problems.

An area which may need further development is the establishment of partnerships among both non-government and government organisations. While project staff occasionally cited examples of engaging with external agencies which could provide complementary expertise, or facilitating exposure visits for staff from other organisations who were interested in learning from and replicating their work, this was the exception rather than the norm. Linkages with government institutions were particularly poor.

Multi-sectoral approaches

Rather than focusing on one area in isolation, all of the projects reviewed are founded on an understanding of the links between HIV/AIDS, poverty, and vulnerability, and respond on a variety of levels. While some projects originated in the health or agricultural sector, over time staff realised the importance of tackling other, wider problems facing PLWHA and their communities, leading to the projects working across sectors. Where this is not possible, staff can make the institutional links necessary to meet wider needs. For example, in the case of one of the projects providing microfinance, the groups established for the distribution of loans became entry points into the community for district government staff and NGOs specialising in social development.

This highlights the importance of an integrated response to the impacts of HIV/AIDS. Even with the advent of new developments (such as access to ARV treatment), interventions that enhance food security, income, and the living conditions of PLWHA and their families will remain critical.

Targeting

In most cases projects do not focus their activities specifically in relation to HIV/AIDS, except for cases of home care and support for PLWHA. Instead, particular categories of people such as resource-poor farmers, women, widows, orphans and those responsible for them, or young people, are the defined beneficiaries, with the assumption that most of these will have been affected to a large extent by HIV/AIDS.

Targeting needs to be handled sensitively, as the success of project interventions very much depends on the responsiveness of the intended beneficiaries. In some cases, attempts to define activities in specific response to the epidemic have faced problems in terms of stigmatisation and resentment within the local community. Furthermore, staff of several projects had experienced situations where PLWHA had refused home care due to the unwanted attention it would draw to their households. It should also be recognised that in a context where people are often unaware of their sero-status, attempting to focus activities on those most immediately affected by HIV/AIDS is often impossible and may not even be advisable. Not all orphans in need are necessarily AIDS orphans, for example, and all children who become heads of household, for whatever reason, require support and protection. Attempting to target livelihood support purely on the basis of a relationship with the epidemic can therefore be artificial. Furthermore, it is not only orphans who face increased hardship – HIV/AIDS has heightened the vulnerability of many young people. Children in households that have taken in a number of dependent relatives, and children who are responsible for caring for sick parents or relatives, are all adversely affected.

Project experiences reveal the importance of understanding and responding to the needs of a whole range of vulnerable groups. What makes some interventions especially innovative and appropriate for AIDS-affected communities is their flexibility to adapt activities for hitherto neglected sectors of the population. Not all of the problems facing these groups are unique to PLWHA or HIV/AIDS-affected communities; in some cases they are continuing problems of poverty. However, it can be seen that HIV/AIDS has exacerbated existing problems and, together with the previous failures of the development process, have left certain individuals and their households even more in need.

Contribution to HIV prevention

One of the known links between HIV/AIDS and poverty is that the impacts of the epidemic can themselves increase the susceptibility of certain social groups to the spread of HIV. For example, women who face economic difficulties and have limited livelihood options (e.g. teenage school dropouts, single mothers, widows) may resort to transactional sex as a means of supplementing income and therefore be at increased risk of HIV infection. Similarly, young people orphaned by AIDS who experience social exclusion in their home communities may migrate from rural to urban areas and are vulnerable to exploitation, which leaves them more exposed to the risk of contracting HIV (UNICEF 2002). By responding to the needs of such groups, livelihood interventions and other efforts to eliminate poverty may play as vital a role in HIV prevention as more conventional activities such as the distribution of condoms.

Impact of HIV/AIDS on the entire human resource base

A further issue which, fortuitously, had not yet affected the interventions reviewed, but of which project staff were certainly aware, was the impact of HIV/AIDS on organisational capacity. Increased absenteeism, staff sickness, and death are now widespread phenomena in every sector, resulting in the loss of experience and skills, growing costs to organisations, and an overall reduction in the capacity to respond to the impacts of HIV/AIDS. New measures, such as supporting staff in gaining access to health care and, in particular, ARV drugs (through staff health-insurance programmes, for example), job sharing, and the mentoring of younger, more inexperienced staff by those with more substantial knowledge and skills, will need to be institutionalised in order to protect organisations from the impacts of HIV/AIDS on their human capital base.

Replicating successful approaches?

The work carried out by NGOs to date reveals how communities affected by HIV/AIDS can be successfully supported in their struggle to combat the consequences of the epidemic. Clearly, greater commitment by donors – whose responses to the epidemic are currently focused on preventive and curative health services – to interventions such as those reviewed could make a significant difference, in terms both of the outreach and the sustainability of such responses. Such a commitment is urgently required.

There is a huge potential for the valuable insights gained from existing project experience to be shared with others who are endeavouring to establish similar initiatives. Information sharing is weak, however, and depends largely on local collaborations and sporadic exchange visits with other local projects. Although a number of information networks (often web-based) are used by project staff, they play a limited role in exchanging experiences. The creation of systematic means of sharing of information could be instrumental not only in ensuring the more effective promotion of successful approaches but also in facilitating the development of new partnerships, a critical and underdeveloped area. The promotion of information networks which reach grassroots practitioners, and the establishment of regular national, regional, and international gatherings aimed at promoting networking and the sharing of experiences could, therefore, play a key role. More systematic and rigorous monitoring and evaluation systems may also need to be instigated across all projects, in order to enable a more structured learning of lessons, and a clearer identification of 'best practice' interventions, an issue which has already been identified (Grainger *et al.* 2001). However, local practitioners may not themselves have the resources, time, or professional skills to carry out these activities. Facilitating the sharing of experiences and the dissemination of lessons learned, and establishing systems for the monitoring and evaluation of progress, may therefore be important roles for external support agencies. All of these activities could make an important contribution to the replication of approaches known to achieve impact.

In many cases project staff are now facing the dilemma of how to increase the impact of their work on a wider scale. Although the concept of 'scaling up' is seductive, a 'one size fits all' approach is unworkable. Experience has revealed the importance of responding to the needs identified by local communities and adapting existing approaches to the particular context in which new work is to be developed. While this is a resource-intensive approach, it is the only means of ensuring that interventions are appropriate and focus on groups most in need of support. This does not, of course, preclude the promotion of successful approaches. Organisations with a proven track record in a particular area could, for example, act as a training resource, in order to facilitate the adaptation of activities that have worked well. This would require external funding support as the capacity-building and resources required would be beyond the current means of most small NGOs.

The replication of successful approaches on a wide scale will require systematic commitment from donors. At the very least, sustained support will be required to ensure that the experiences of those at the forefront of the struggle to combat the impacts of the epidemic are shared both regionally and internationally.[4]

Conclusions

The NGO responses to HIV/AIDS in sub-Saharan Africa summarised in this chapter demonstrate the potential range of multi-sectoral interventions which can be undertaken in order to support vulnerable groups, such as women, orphans, and young people, who are bearing the brunt of the epidemic. The promotion of appropriate technologies for agricultural production, skills training, strategic income-generation activities, and the provision of credit, are approaches which are already being seen to have made a difference to AIDS-affected communities.

A major challenge is the introduction of appropriate monitoring and evaluation systems and wider sharing of experiences and lessons so that similar activities are promoted as a matter of urgency. Efforts also need to be made to ensure that donors increase the funding made available for initiatives to mitigate the impacts of HIV/AIDS. It is therefore critical that rigorous analyses of experiences and achievements to date are carefully disseminated to donor agencies as well as to other practitioners.

This article was originally published in Development in Practice, *volume 15, number 2, March 2005.*

Acknowledgements

The project review detailed in this paper was funded by DFID under the Advisory and Support Services Commission for the benefit of developing countries. The views expressed are not necessarily those of DFID. See White (2002) for details of the full report.

References

Allen, H. (2002) 'CARE International's Village Savings and Loan Programmes in Africa: Micro-finance for the Rural Poor that Works', unpublished report, Dar es Salaam: CARE International.

Baylies, C. (2002) 'The impact of AIDS on rural households in Africa: a shock like any other?', *Development and Change* 33(4): 611–32.

De Waal, A. (2002) '"New variant famine" in Southern Africa', unpublished paper for SADC VAC Meeting, Victoria Falls, 17–18 October.

Donahue, J. (1999) 'Microfinance and Community Mobilization as HIV/AIDS Mitigation Tools', prepared for the Displaced Children and Orphans fund of USAID as a supplementary report to *Children Affected by HIV/AIDS in Kenya: An Overview of Issues and Action to Strengthen Community Care and Support,* Washington, DC: Displaced Children and Orphans Fund/USAID and UNICEF.

Donahue, J., K. Kabbucho, and S. Osinde (2001) *HIV/AIDS – Responding to a Silent Crisis among Microfinance Clients in Kenya and Uganda*, Nairobi: MicroSave-Africa.

Grainger, C., D. Webb, and L. Elliott (2001) 'Children Affected by HIV/AIDS: Rights and Responses in the Developing World', Save the Children Working Paper 23, London: Save the Children UK.

UNAIDS (2002) *Report on the Global HIV/AIDS Epidemic*, Geneva: UNAIDS.

UNAIDS/WHO (2003) 'AIDS Epidemic Update', available at www.unaids.org

UNICEF (2002) *Orphans and Other Children Affected by HIV/AIDS: A UNICEF Fact Sheet*, New York: UNICEF.

Villareal, M. (2002) 'Perspective: How Can Agriculture Face the Challenges Posed by HIV/AIDS?', *NewAgriculturalist online*, available at www.new-agri.co.uk/02-5/perspect.html (last accessed August 2007).

White, J. (2002) 'Facing the Challenge: NGO Responses to the Impacts of HIV/AIDS', unpublished report, Chatham: Natural Resources Institute, University of Greenwich, available at www.nri.org/news/pdfaidsreport nov2002.pdf (last accessed August 2007).

White, J. and E. Robinson (2000) *HIV/AIDS and Rural Livelihoods in Sub-Saharan Africa*, NRI Policy Series No. 6, Chatham: Natural Resources Institute, University of Greenwich.

World Bank (1997) *Confronting AIDS – Public Priorities in a Global Epidemic*, Oxford: Oxford University Press.

Notes

1 See www.livelihoods.org for further information concerning the diverse range of livelihood activities on which rural communities in sub-Saharan Africa rely.

2 This view was expressed by a number of government representatives who attended an FAO Technical Meeting, December 2001.

3 This is particularly important in an environment where there is limited medical support. At the time of writing, none of the projects reviewed was involved in facilitating access to ARV drugs for the treatment of HIV/AIDS.

4 Since the preparation of this chapter, there have been several donor-supported meetings focused on HIV/AIDS, agriculture, and livelihoods. See, for example, www.sarpn.org.za/mitigation_of_HIV_AIDS, the web page of a 2003 conference on the mitigation of the impacts of HIV/AIDS on agriculture and rural development.

10 Danger and opportunity: responding to HIV with vision

Kate Butcher and Alice Welbourn

Among trainers in participatory approaches to development, there is a legendary indigenous language which uses one character to represent the concepts of both 'danger' and 'opportunity'. This symbol, which simultaneously represents two very different attitudes to a situation, reminds us of different ways in which people have responded to HIV/AIDS. HIV has now been an issue of major concern for at least 20 years and continues to pose immense challenges, which humanity has been unable to meet. Yet many individuals and groups who are infected with HIV, or touched in other ways, have risen to its challenge. One key example is Noerine Kaleeba, who founded TASO in Uganda in 1986 (Hampton 1990). We feel that development workers owe it to extraordinary people like Noerine to consider what opportunities may be presented by the danger of HIV.

The difference between the agendas of health personnel and other development professionals and those groups who are targeted for their attention has been a problematic aspect of much HIV work in the past. Most have set their own agendas in response to HIV, and have developed an 'us and them' approach, focusing mainly on prevention work among groups of people who are viewed as 'vulnerable groups' and from whom workers can distinguish themselves clearly. Sex workers are one such example. However, some programmes and projects have taken a much wider approach, contextualising the health issues inherent in HIV within their social context. Below, we give some examples of such innovative work.

The Working Women's Project: understanding people's own priorities

In Bradford, a city in the north of England, the Working Women's Project was established in early 1991, in response to growing public concerns about HIV. Public funds for the Bradford project were earmarked for 'HIV', and the project was ostensibly conceived to reduce infections within the population of sex workers and beyond. It was widely assumed by the health service and the local authority that in order to stop the spread of HIV infection in the UK population, sex workers (who sometimes refer to themselves as 'working women') should be targeted for HIV education. Of course, as with so many similar projects, it did not take long to establish that sexual health was not a high-priority issue for many of the sex workers. Their priorities were, rather, to avoid arrest by the police and violence from clients, police, and pimps; to care for their families; and to achieve economic solvency. Health was at the bottom of their list. It is unsurprising that sex workers in many other parts of the world share these same priorities.

Responding to the views and agendas of groups 'targeted' for development work necessitates moving beyond a narrow focus on a project, to concentrate on attitudes and approaches. In Bradford, HIV prevention was the agenda of the health authority, and not of the women. As project workers, our job was to navigate the grey waters in between. In Bradford, establishing credibility with the sex workers themselves, and building a project which went some way to meet their needs, involved many years of listening and responding. After the first year, a group of women approached the project staff (of whom Kate Butcher was one) to say that they were heartily sick of reading articles about 'prostitutes', which bore no or little relation to their own experience.

Collectively, it was decided that those women interested would contribute their experiences to a book, which would not be edited in a way which integrated a social analysis, but would rather be a stand-alone book of testimonies 'in our own words', whose contents could therefore neither be refuted or approved: it was simply to be a collection of their own stories in their own words. The book took over two years to produce. It was pulled together from very loosely structured interviews with 11 women. Each chapter begins with a poem written by one of the sex workers, and the final poem is a contribution by a client. The process of putting the book together was an empowering one; women began to see points of commonality in their lives, rather than issues which encouraged competition between them. It was agreed among them that the book should be dedicated to the three women who had died during the first two years of the project, two as a result of violence and one from a drug overdose. It was a powerful reminder of the centrality of violence in sex workers' lives. Those who contributed to the book came together again over a year later, to organise a memorial service for one of their friends who was murdered on the street. Obviously, this was a tragic and traumatic time, but the sex workers were determined to make their voices heard. There is no magic formula to guarantee the success of such an activity, simply the willingness of those employed to work with different communities to listen to people, and to respect them as equals.

The concept of sharing experiences with women was critical to the success of the Working Women's Project. Kate Butcher went on to work in Nepal in a different capacity, but continued her links with sex-work projects. During this time, she ran a workshop with sex workers in Kathmandu for the British Council (Butcher and White 1997). The workshop was designed to help women to identify their major concerns about their work and then to share and develop coping strategies. The common issues of concern to both sets of women were far removed from the HIV-prevention agenda of the professional health staff in their respective countries. As key issues in their lives, the 30 Nepalese sex workers clearly identified violence at work and at home, and intimidation and violence from the police. There was a deep-rooted commonality in the collective experiences of these women from Bradford and Kathmandu. At the end of the week, Kate Butcher invited women to use a hand-held video camera, to send messages to sister sex workers in the UK. They were encouraged to ask questions. They asked about the rates that women charged for their work in Bradford, and recounted their own stories of arrest, or strategies for avoiding violence or police harassment. When the video was shown in Bradford, the women there could scarcely believe the similarity to their own experiences. (They were also amazed that anyone could actually 'do business' in a sari!)

It was only by addressing and recognising the issues fundamental to women's lives that we were subsequently able to go on to work with them on the issues of HIV prevention and improved sexual health. In a sense, we ended up with a reciprocal arrangement between project workers and the women themselves, in which we acknowledged the importance of violence or housing or children in their lives, and they in turn acknowledged the importance of achieving and maintaining a good level of sexual health.

Supporting positive people in their response to HIV

In the past, health and development workers have often viewed people with HIV and those perceived as 'at risk' as objects of blame, or, at best, of pity. Most agencies have assumed that once people are HIV-positive, they are really a lost cause.[1] There are a few notable exceptions who have focused on care and support for those who have HIV, and even fewer who have viewed HIV-positive people, or others in marginalised groups seen as 'at risk', as equal actors who can play a central role in responding positively to the challenge of HIV.

There have been many responses from people living with HIV to negative attitudes towards their condition, including a great frustration with judgemental, insensitive, and irrelevant approaches from health workers. For example, in 1998, the International Community of Women Living with HIV, an NGO founded in 1992,[2] launched its own research project to study the needs and perspectives of positive women, called Voices and Choices (Feldman *et al.*, 2006). In Zimbabwe, positive women from many different backgrounds worked together with other women on the steering group, underwent training in interview techniques, and developed their own set of questions for the research project. From work with groups of positive women all over Zimbabwe, key findings included initial reactions of blame and anger from family members; the huge loss of income faced by positive people and their families from loss of property and labour, through both stigma and ill health; lack of access to health care and children's education through poverty and stigma; lack of access to information about *living* with HIV; social expectations which made women powerless to gain access to or use condoms; fears about infecting children; and the impact on widows of male-biased inheritance laws. The women commented that they had gained huge support from other positive women in local peer groups, and that the development of counselling services had also helped them to begin to address some issues concerning unequal gender relations with their husbands. For the most part, however, although HIV-prevention information was widespread, it had never seemed relevant to them before their diagnosis, since they had not seen themselves as being at particular risk of infection.[3] They said information had not given them the tools to address any of the issues with their own partners, either before or since.

Since conducting the Voices and Choices research, many of the HIV-positive women involved have developed the self-confidence to join local health committees, have engaged in public speaking, and have attended workshops on gender violence and other related matters. They have also networked with other relevant groups in Zimbabwe. The experiences of the positive women of Zimbabwe echo the concerns of the sex workers of Nepal and Bradford, raised earlier. They touch on issues of poverty, violence, and stigma; of a wish for children; of lack of choice – a reflection of the huge range of issues relating to gender and poverty which were in existence for many years before the advent of HIV. Now, ironically, HIV is itself becoming such a great threat to health and life that funding is available and there is a preparedness to begin to address these sensitive (often taboo) issues in ways which never before existed.

Nurturing alternative views: involving men in HIV-support services

While gender-related issues affecting women have been a key and growing concern for development and social policy, the resultant programmes and policies have often failed to get to the heart of the problem, which is rooted in intimate relationships between women and men. Transforming the relationships between women and men demands attention to male gender identity, and the role of men in preventing violence and promoting reproductive health. Attention must also be paid to the achievement of other social goals, including responsible parenting. One particular area of taboo for men is the need for them to be engaged in the process of challenging gender-based inequality and gender stereotypes. Men need to be engaged, partly because of their role within families as gatekeepers (if they were not themselves involved and did not agree to the discussions, they could ban their wives from attending discussions about women's roles – and beat them if they disobeyed), but also because they have their own gender-related concerns and needs in terms of sexual health. Although those working in the field of gender have for many years known and struggled with the need to involve men in gender analysis, and the development of gender-aware policy and practice, there is now an increasing international awareness among (largely male-dominated) senior NGO staff (and large donors too) of the importance of sound gender-based work with men in the fight against HIV. The example below, from Brazil, illustrates how this can be done.

Promundo is an NGO working in the *favelas*[4] of Rio de Janeiro, Brazil (Barker 2001). Its activities include work on gender inequality, health, and issues facing adolescents; prevention of intra-personal violence, including gender-based violence; and provision of support to families living with HIV. Promundo has developed an action-research project to work with young men in a context where domestic violence is widely seen as normal behaviour: a powerful image of manhood for these young men. Women are popularly viewed as sexual objects who must always be faithful, whereas men are entitled to have occasional sexual relationships with other women. Links between domestic and sexual violence are also related to unemployment, a history of physical violence in childhood, and a prevailing silence among men about the violence which they see around them.

When the project was still in its research phase, Promundo staff realised that there were often one or two young men in a discussion group who viewed the world differently, and had the self-confidence to question in front of their peers the established view that violence against women was justifiable in order for men to maintain control over their behaviour. Promundo then developed ways of working with these few young men, helping them to analyse the background of violence in their lives and to explore alternative, more positive ways of behaviour. Some older men, who had already formed a group called 'Male Consciousness', were invited to collaborate in the work, acting as positive role models for the younger men. The latter, in turn, were hired as peer promoters.

The peer promoters and other young men wove their own personal stories into a play and a photo novella, entitled *Cool Your Head Man*. The play, which explores relationships, domestic violence, and health issues, is currently presented widely around the *favelas*, and the photo novella is distributed among the audiences. The photo novella enjoins men to 'reflect before they act, and to cool down when they are angry, rather than use violence'. This project is only in its infancy, but through engaging with these young men, their partners, parents, and opinion leaders, it is beginning to build on those few exceptions to the norm which already existed, to explore different ways of viewing violence in the community. The project is based on the recognition that there is a long way to go to challenge ingrained attitudes to gender relations and violence, but that, through building on existing awareness and through encouraging the development of local materials and performances, a sense of local ownership of the project can be built, which will enable its success to spread.

Working from different starting points: Stepping Stones

Another programme which takes a wider approach to HIV than the narrow health-focused model is Stepping Stones, a training package designed for community-wide use (Welbourn 1995). Initially produced as a resource for rural communities in sub-Saharan Africa, with a strong emphasis on HIV and gender issues, it has now been successfully adapted and translated by various organisations, in many different contexts (Gordon and Phiri 2000).

These local adaptations have been a key part of the success of Stepping Stones. This is because, although the package covers many different issues (such as responses to the use of alcohol; patterns of access to and control of money in the household; gender-based violence; ways of building self-esteem, assertiveness and effective communication skills; and even preparing for death), the central focus of the original manual was HIV. However, as we have tried to show above, HIV is normally not the issue at the front of the minds of the people with whom we may be trying to work. This is true even of people in countries with a high prevalence of HIV, such as Uganda. For instance, after a Stepping Stones workshop there, young women reported that they were now able to negotiate condom use and were glad that they could do so, because it would protect them from … *pregnancy*. They were more immediately fearful of being expelled from school because of pregnancy than of contracting HIV (personal experience 1996). It follows from this that, if international funders rush in to promote their concerns about HIV (especially in countries where the prevalence – at least officially – is still low), there is a great chance of doing more harm than good.

As an alternative approach, programmes run by the Planned Parenthood Association of South Africa and the South African Medical Research Council Women's Health Unit in South Africa (Jewkes *et al.* 2000), and in Gambia by the Gambian Family Planning Association, the British Medical Research Council, ActionAid, and others, have successfully adapted Stepping Stones to suit local concerns by presenting the package as a fertility-protection programme (Shaw and Jawo 2000). People in both these countries, one with high HIV prevalence, one with still relatively low HIV prevalence, are anxious to maintain their fertility. In Gambia, a polygamous society, there were also fears that Stepping Stones was yet another Western-inspired population-control programme.[5] By presenting Stepping Stones as a programme which will enable couples to have children when they want to do so, as well as protect themselves from the STIs which often cause infertility, staff have successfully developed the package in a manner which has been well received.[6] By starting off with what concerns participants most, facilitators have been able to earn their trust, which has in turn enabled them to go on to address other related issues.

In the programmes of both countries, as elsewhere in contexts in which Stepping Stones has been well adapted and well facilitated, participants have identified the positive outcomes as a reduction in gender violence, increased sharing of household expenditure, an increase in condom use, reduced alcohol consumption, more equitable inheritance, more satisfaction in sexual relations, and a reduced number of sexual partners (Welbourn 1999).[7] The staff in the programmes concerned also comment that it is now possible to find words to talk about issues which until now have been entirely taboo subjects.

It is ironic that, so much money having been spent on population-*reduction* strategies over the past 20 years, an approach to HIV/AIDS-prevention which can be presented as a fertility-protection strategy should now show signs of achieving so much. Once more, work on HIV seems to be teaching development and community workers – at last – the importance of beginning with local people's own agendas, rather than with their own.

Supporting traditional service-providers

Another arena where HIV might be beginning to make a difference is the care and support of sick people. Women have long been seen by gender analysts as 'triple providers', in their productive and reproductive roles, and as community maintenance workers. In caring at home for loved ones who are sick, women yet again bear the brunt of the workload. Pioneering organisations have evolved, offering support to positive people, such as TASO in Uganda (Hampton 1990) and Chikankata in Zambia (Williams 1990). In the mid-1980s, these courageously began to care for people with HIV and AIDS and their families, and provide non-judgemental support services. At that time, their approach was unique. Yet even these organisations, and those which followed their example, have still done little to challenge the traditional gender models which represent women as the sole providers of such support.

However, signs of change are beginning to appear. In Cambodia, for instance, KHANA, the Khmer HIV/AIDS NGO Alliance, is now working with men, not only to raise their awareness of HIV and their role in prevention, but also to promote their role in providing care for the sick. 'Men have a crucial role to play...and the LNGOs are beginning to work with men in their local communities to identify strategies to do so. Peer group discussions raise awareness of issues such as discrimination and human rights and explore the role men can play in meeting care and support needs in the community.' (Sellers *et al.* 2006)

The advent of HIV has also raised awareness among development workers of the key role which traditional community healers have to play, both spiritually and physically, in care and support of people with all kinds of problems. While most development workers in the past have kept well clear of traditional healers, believing that their own role was to promote a narrow Western biomedical model of health care, some others have begun to work with traditional healers to promote a more holistic approach to HIV. In Uganda in 1992, one innovative group of traditional healers and doctors joined hands to form a new group called THETA (Traditional and Modern Health Practitioners Together Against AIDS). Displaying mutual respect, trust, and a spirit of openness on both sides, they worked hard to overcome more conventional rivalries and hostilities (Kaleeba *et al.* 2000).

THETA first conducted a study of the efficacy of certain traditional herbs for treating problems common among HIV-positive people, such as herpes zoster and chronic diarrhoea. There were marked improvements in the health of those involved in the study. Subsequently, a second project developed, called THEWA (Traditional Healers, Women and AIDS Prevention), which developed a gender-sensitive, culturally appropriate strategy for educating and counselling people about HIV/AIDS. Out of this then grew a third initiative, which trained healers from eight districts in Uganda as HIV-prevention educators and counsellors. The training sessions, based on the participatory skills in which the trainers themselves had been trained, proved very popular.

An evaluation of THETA in 1997–98 showed some major changes in traditional healers' knowledge of and attitudes towards HIV, their ability to share this knowledge with others, their capacity to counsel others, and their readiness to promote condom use. One spiritualist healer explained: 'We requested our ancestral spirits to understand the serious situation we are in, and they have allowed us to talk about condoms and to promote condoms.' Referrals from traditional healers to Western health-service providers, and *vice versa*, now take place regularly, as each group of providers grows to recognise the limitations of its own services, and the scope of the other's skills. Traditional healers have also supported the development of positive people's own support groups. Above all, they have helped positive people, their families, and communities to cope better with the impact of HIV and to reduce its spread.

Changing attitudes through working with authorities

While providing and facilitating communal, spiritual, and physical support are all crucial elements of a positive response to HIV, the case studies of the Bradford and Nepalese sex workers, and the HIV-positive women in Zimbabwe also reveal their fear of the authorities. The sex workers were concerned about police harassment; the positive women in Zimbabwe were concerned about laws which favour male inheritance systems. Some organisations have adopted strategies to change the attitudes of the authorities, and challenge the discriminatory rules and systems over which they have jurisdiction.

The Musasa Project, a far-sighted and enterprising NGO in Zimbabwe that works to eradicate violence against women, began to work with the police and the judiciary in 1988, with the objective of fostering a greater understanding of the 'rape culture' and tolerance of domestic violence that Musasa argues exists in Zimbabwe (Stewart 1996). Few Zimbabwean women dared to report incidents of violence against them, because women often blamed themselves for these attacks, and the police and members of the judiciary often added to this sense of blame through their insensitive and accusatory responses. Musasa managed to work closely with the police and judiciary to develop new, more private reporting processes which were both quicker and more sensitive to the women's needs. A faster, simpler approach to the whole system was developed with the police, to bring the accused to court, treat what the women said seriously, and prosecute rapists. Musasa highlights the close collaboration with the authorities as a key part of its success. Since those early years, Musasa has developed to do further work with victims of domestic violence.

While Musasa's work did not specifically arise out of an aim to respond to HIV, it now also works closely with organisations such as WASN (discussed earlier), in a collaborative response to HIV. It has begun to focus on the entire range of activities related to HIV and STIs, including counselling and legal services, public education, and advocacy work.[8]

'Mainstreaming' responses to HIV into the work of development agencies

As HIV continues to wreak havoc in the poorest parts of the world, it has taken too long for development workers to recognise that the impact of HIV and AIDS extends far beyond the areas of concern of the formal health sector: the illness and deaths of large parts of the population – including young and middle-aged adults in the prime of their productive years – result in social and economic fragmentation of society. In many ways, the most acute challenges are yet to come, because the time-lag between infection and eventual illness is long, and the enormity of the problem in some parts of the world – for example, South Asia and Eastern Europe – is only now becoming obvious. However, particularly in areas of the world where HIV took root sooner, the social and economic impact of HIV on livelihoods and all other aspects of human life is now evident.

Consequently, many more development workers are now becoming engaged in thinking and planning which integrates HIV-awareness into all aspects of their work. In particular, they are considering ways of communicating the messages about prevention to as many people as possible in as many ways as possible. 'Mainstreaming' HIV offers an opportunity to address a range of issues which seem to fall through the cracks of standard development work: namely how people relate to each other at work and at home, and how destructive situations can be changed for the good of all. No longer the preserve of formal-sector health workers or health promoters designing their information, education, and communication (IEC) campaigns, HIV-awareness is being mainstreamed into all development activities in a welcome – if tardy – recognition that it is not only people who attend clinics who are vulnerable to HIV, or put others at risk. An opportunity is now opening up to address the issues of inter-personal relationships which have always been a problem, and have always had an impact on people's social and economic well-being, no matter whether there is a high or low prevalence of HIV.

Recently, a training workshop was developed for technical staff and administrators employed by the UK government's Department for International Development (DFID), in an effort to update all workers' understanding of HIV and AIDS and to help them to work through the issues which it raises in the workplace (Butcher and Butler 2000). The workshop has been conducted for several departments of DFID in the UK, and also in some of its overseas offices, including those in Nigeria, Pakistan, and India. The package was designed largely to help advisers and technical staff – both British and national – to think more creatively about their work and to identify areas in which they may be able to contribute to the fight against AIDS, whether in the workplace, or through their development programmes in sectors such as health, education, and governance. The workshop provides participants with opportunities to explore the broader implications of HIV, both personally and professionally.

In Pakistan, a country with an apparently low prevalence of HIV, the participants on the workshop course were mostly administrative workers from the UK Foreign Office, working at a local level. They had little responsibility for the development of DFID's programme. Initially, it was felt that the outcomes of the day might be hampered by lack of input from a programme perspective. However, this was not the case. By concentrating in a gender-sensitive and non-threatening environment on what mattered to the participants, other issues were raised which we had overlooked. For instance, one woman mentioned her relief at attending the workshop, which was giving her a better understanding of the epidemic, but also voiced her concern that she would have to talk about HIV with her prospective husband. She wondered how could she do that, in a society where sex is not openly discussed between women and men. Another woman mentioned rape and the concomitant threat of becoming infected. Regarding workplace issues, the two-day session pointed out clearly the responsibility of the employer to provide a confidential and competent counselling service to all employees who may require it. Happily, at the end of the mission two independent external counsellors were identified, and DFID plans to make their skills available to its employees (and their partners, if they wish).

Domestic violence and emotional stress had already been noted as having an impact on work performance, but they had not been addressed in any clear way before. The HIV workshop allowed a frank exchange of ideas and provided an opportunity for participants to discuss these issues. As a result we were able to identify referral points for staff seeking support, whether their concerns were directly connected with HIV or with relationships in general. DFID has now adopted an internal plan to 'continue to raise awareness among staff of HIV/AIDS issues, including their own vulnerability to HIV', and to address care and support issues for staff with HIV (DFID 2001).

Conclusion

It is promising that development organisations, including large international NGOs and major bilateral donors, are now starting to encourage their own staff to make the links between their professional and personal lives, so that at last barriers between 'us and them', which have for so long prevented the acknowledgement of the impact of HIV on the lives of *all* of us, may be removed. There is a danger here that traditional approaches to HIV may be developed as an after-thought to existing projects, such as engineering, water, or forestry projects. The corresponding opportunity is to build on the lessons offered by innovative approaches, like the ones we have described here. Lack of space prevents us from describing many more kinds of intervention – for example, work with religious leaders, with older women on female initiation, with men who have sex with men, or with people in same-sex relationships.

Overall, we have gained from these innovations a greater appreciation of the following needs:

- To involve, whenever possible, the people who are the focus of development and community work, and their loved ones, in the planning and development of needs-based responses. In this article, we have given examples of sex workers, young men, rape survivors, development-agency staff, and HIV-positive people. Whoever they may be, they need to be involved.

- To engage men, as well as women, in the response, in reflection of their traditional roles as gatekeepers, as well as their own sexual and reproductive health needs.

- To develop a gender-aware response which addresses the strategic needs of women and the benefits to both women and men of more equitable access to and control of material goods and services; to engage local people in local production of their own communication materials, in order to ensure a local sense of ownership of the changes they wish to see.

- To develop responses to HIV/AIDS not only in countries where HIV prevalence is already known to be high, but in countries with low prevalence, to keep it that way. This is in recognition of the links between poor sexual health and domestic violence, gender inequalities, and poverty which are already prevalent in many countries.

We have tried to highlight the need for a collaborative, multi-layered response to HIV/AIDS from the development community, from bilateral agencies and civil-society organisations together, both internationally and nationally. This response needs to take place at many levels: at community level, through traditional and formal-sector service provision, through religious and political leadership, through workplace support, and through legal guarantees of the human rights of HIV-positive people and their families. A truly multi-sectoral response is needed, which fully addresses the diversity of causes and consequences of HIV infection. HIV is here now, and there is no more time to lose. By building on the lessons we have already learned we can save time – and lives.

This article was originally published in Gender & Development, *volume 9, number 2, July 2001.*

References

Barker, G. (2001) '"Cool your head, man": Results from an action-research initiative to engage young men in preventing gender-based violence in favelas in Rio de Janeiro, Brazil', *Development* 44(3): 94–8.

Butcher, K. and A. Butler (2000) 'Mainstreaming HIV', unpublished paper, John Snow International UK.

Butcher, K. and S. Chapple (1996) *Doing Business*, Bradford Health Authority.

Butcher, K. and K. White (1997) 'Women's empowerment training', *British Council Network Newsletter* no. 14.

DFID (2001) *HIV/AIDS Strategy*. Available at www.dfid.gov.uk.

Feldman, R., J. Manchester, and C. Maposhere (2006) 'Positive women: voices and choices in Zimbabwe', in A. Cornwall and A. Welbourn (eds.), *Realizing Rights: Transforming Approaches to Sexual and Reproductive Well-being*, London: Zed Books.

Gangakhedkar, Raman R., M. E. Bentley, A. D. Divekar, *et al.* (1997) 'Spread of HIV infection in married monogamous women in India', *Journal of the American Medical Association*, 278 (23).

Gordon, G. and F. Phiri (2000) 'Moving beyond the "KAP GAP": a community based reproductive health programme in Eastern Province, Zambia', in A. Cornwall and A. Welbourn (eds.), *From Reproduction to Rights: Participatory Approaches to Sexual and Reproductive Health*, PLA Notes 37, London: IIED.

Hampton, J. (1990) *Living Positively with AIDS: The AIDS Support Organization*, Strategies for Hope no. 2, London: ActionAid.

Jewkes, R., C. Matubatuba, D. Metsing, E. Ngcobo, F. Makaota, G. Mbhalati, J. Frohlich, K. Wood, K. Kabi, L. Ncube, N. Nduna, N. Jama, P. Moumakoe, and S. Raletsemo (2000) *Stepping Stones: Feedback from the Field*. Available at: www.stratshope.org/feedback.html.

Kaleeba, N., J. N. Kadowe, D. Kalinaki, and G. Williams (eds.) (2000) *Open Secret: People facing up to HIV and AIDS in Uganda*, Strategies for Hope no. 15, London: ActionAid.

Sellers, T., P. Panhavichetr, L. Chansophal, and A. Maclean (2006) 'Promoting the participation of men in community-based HIV/AIDS prevention and care in Cambodia', in A. Cornwall and A. Welbourn (eds.), *Realizing Rights: Transforming Approaches to Sexual and Reproductive Well-being*, London: Zed Books.

Shaw, M. and M. Jawo (2000) 'Gambian experiences with Stepping Stones: 1996–9', in A. Cornwall and A. Welbourn (eds.), *From Reproduction to Rights: Participatory Approaches to Sexual and Reproductive Health*, PLA Notes 37, London: IIED.

Stewart, S. (1996) 'Changing attitudes towards violence against women: the Musasa Project', in Zeidenstein and Moore (eds.), *Learning about Sexuality: A Practical Beginning*, New York: Population Council.

Welbourn, A. (1995) *Stepping Stones: A Training Package on HIV, Communication and Relationship Skills,* Strategies for Hope, London: ActionAid.

Welbourn, A. (1999) 'Gender, Sex and HIV: how to address issues that no-one wants to hear about', paper presented at the Geneva Symposium: 'Tant qu'on a la santé', Geneva: DDC, UNESCO, and IUED.

Williams, G. (1990) *From Fear to Hope: AIDS Care and Prevention at Chikankata Hospital, Zambia*, Strategies for Hope no.1, London: ActionAid.

Notes

1 USAID, for instance, has only recently started to fund care programmes.

2 ICW was established in 1992 by HIV-positive women from 27 countries in response to the lack of support and information available to women diagnosed with HIV infection.

3 This echoes research from India which found that the highest rate of increase in HIV infection was among married monogamous women, who never thought themselves to be at risk of HIV (Gangakhedkar *et al.*1997).

4 Urban slum areas.

5 AIDS is often known in Africa as 'American Initiative to Discourage Sex'.

6 The Stepping Stones Gambia Adaptation has just been adopted by the government of Gambia as a nationwide community-based initiative.

7 There are local Stepping Stones adaptations and translations in use both in Africa and Asia. See: www.stratshope.org/t-languages.htm (last accessed August 2007).

8 For more recent information about Musasa see, for example: www.qweb.kvinnoforum.se/members/musasa.html.

11 'Mainstreaming' HIV in Papua New Guinea: putting gender equity first

Janet Seeley and Kate Butcher

The travel guide books (Lonely Planet 2005) talk of Papua New Guinea (PNG) as 'a raw land, remarkably untamed and as variegated as swamp and jagged limestone' and warn the traveller about crime, banditry, and violence. The warnings to the traveller are not misplaced, yet it is not just the traveller who needs to take care: violence is a reality with which many Papua New Guineans live all the time (Windybank and Manning 2003). Seventy per cent of women have experienced domestic violence, according to a 1998 World Bank study (Brouwer *et al.* 1998). Such levels of violence are unacceptable in themselves, but this violence is also playing a part in fuelling a rapidly growing HIV epidemic in the country. While evidence as to the extent of the epidemic is still limited (World Bank 2004), it is becoming apparent that the same factors that fuel the epidemic elsewhere in the developing world are at play in PNG; namely, poor infrastructure and lack of accessible services, high poverty and social deprivation, and high rates of partner exchange, together with the increasing mobility of people from rural areas to towns. Gender inequality has an important part to play in the epidemic; the status of women is extremely low in many of the 800 culture groups on the islands, and there is a high level of gender violence and abuse (Yawa n.d.).

The Medium Term Development Strategy (MTDS) 2005–2010 of the government of PNG sets out its overarching development strategy as 'export-driven economic growth, rural development and poverty reduction ...The strategy will be realised by empowering Papua New Guineans, especially those in rural areas, to mobilise their own resources for higher living standards' (Government of PNG 2004, iii). The MTDS identifies the need to develop infrastructure, and improve health and education services.

Included in the MTDS is a list of serious threats to its success. HIV is the first on that list, recognising that the epidemic, which is rapidly worsening in PNG, can undermine all development efforts (*ibid.*). Gender inequality is listed as a constraint that has been recognised since PNG gained independence in 1975. It is stated in the MTDS that gender inequality 'continues to be a key focus of the MTDS 2005–2010' (*ibid.*, 8). The authors refer to 'male gender issues' as well as 'female gender issues', acknowledging that to address gender inequality means looking at issues around men and masculine identities (*ibid.*, 26). A direct link between HIV and gender inequality is not made.

Opportunities to link initiatives aiming to 'mainstream HIV' in development with those intended to 'mainstream gender' are not always seized, partly because the two activities may be undertaken by different people, or because separate programmes and budget lines force a distinction to be made. Indeed, the view that 'mainstreaming' is a separate vertical activity may mean that the idea of mainstreaming more than one concern at a time might just seem too difficult![1] This is because mainstreaming is frequently perceived as a specific programme of activities. Funds for HIV-related activities continue to grow in PNG; the country has just been awarded almost $30 million from the Global Fund to Fight AIDS, Tuberculosis and Malaria for the HIV response. In this context, as elsewhere, 'HIV and AIDS' are increasingly being seen as a sector in their own right. In contrast, the philosophy of mainstreaming HIV advocates 'a process of adapting core business to cope with the realities of HIV and AIDS' (Butcher 2003, 4).

In this article, we argue that the situation in PNG illustrates very clearly not only the need to 'mainstream HIV' into the core business of development, but also that mainstreaming HIV cannot happen without mainstreaming gender. Now, more than ever, greater efforts are needed across the development spectrum to identify and document practices that improve women's status in order to ascertain whether or not these improvements change the dynamics of the epidemic. If they do, it is essential to promote the wider adoption of such practices. In addition, it is also important that those advocating HIV mainstreaming learn from and work with what has been, and is still being, done to promote gender mainstreaming.[2]

This chapter draws on an example from the oil-palm industry in PNG, and suggests that this exemplifies how an initiative developed to address gender inequality has the potential for halting the spread of HIV, and can be adapted further to counter the impact of HIV on families. Before discussing the initiative, however, the next section briefly looks at gender relations and the status of women in PNG.

The HIV and AIDS context in PNG

PNG has an estimated population of five and a half million people. A recent consensus workshop estimated a median of 1.7 per cent HIV prevalence in the adult population (National AIDS Council 2004). PNG has the highest reported rate of HIV infection in the Pacific (UNAIDS/UNICEF/WHO 2004) but the exact number of people infected at this time is unknown. There were 10,184 confirmed cases in September 2004,[3] but this figure masks the fact that many people have not been tested, and data, particularly from rural areas, are unreliable. What is clear is that the total number of people infected is very likely to be much higher than the reported and confirmed cases, with the most recent estimates (2005) of the total number of people living with HIV varying from under 50,000 to over 80,000 (Dugue 2004).

Most of those known to be infected are aged 15 to 34 years, with the largest number of reported cases being among women aged 20 to 24 years (World Bank 2004). This generalised epidemic is heterosexual in nature and, as in many countries in Africa, women are coming to be more severely affected than men (UNAIDS 2004). In addition, PNG has the dubious reputation for having the highest rates of sexually transmitted infections in the region (Mgone *et al.* 2002; Passey *et al.* 1998).

Although the cultural diversity of PNG makes generalisations difficult and unwise, the literature consistently records that women throughout PNG have less access to health care and education than men, have relatively heavier workloads, and are, as noted above, vulnerable to sexual violence. Maternal mortality rates are among the highest in the world, and women's participation in local government is between three per cent and nine per cent. Women make up only 18 per cent of the formal labour force, and hold only 12 per cent of management positions (Asian Development Bank 2002). Despite constitutional and legal provisions, women still often face discrimination. Violence against women (including domestic violence and gang – or 'pack' – rape) affects the day-to-day lives of all women in PNG (Yawa n.d.). PNG is, in the words of an Asian Development Bank review, 'a man's world' (p. 4) particularly in the highlands where 'the dominance and high status of men [are] in contrast to the submission and low status of women' (Yawa n.d.). In many places, men exert control over women's fertility, labour, and freedom of movement. A World Bank report concluded that 'the rights of kinsmen to chastise and punish women were pervasive, and the majority of men and women in PNG still uphold many of men's rights over women' (Brouwer *et al.* 1998, 11).

The age and gender balance in villages has been affected by two factors. First is the loss of young (and sometimes older) men from the rural areas, who go in search of work in the towns. Second is the temporary migration of men to work on plantations. This has led to women, who are responsible for the majority of food crop production, taking on 'male' agricultural tasks such as clearing bush and the cultivation of cash crops (such as coffee) (Gustafsson 2002; Newlin 2000). Women who were already busy thus end up with more to do. Yet the absence of men and the taking on of their tasks has positive benefits for women's roles and authority, as it can be seen that they are able to take on such work. Male out-migration has a negative side when returning men object to women's new-found authority in the home. They may also return with sexually transmitted diseases contracted in the towns, where men greatly outnumber women.

In areas such as the highlands of PNG, where patrilineal systems of inheritance prevail, women's lack of direct control over land limits their ability to undertake cash cropping in their own right. This is because local cultural practice was reinforced by colonial attitudes that prevented women from acquiring blocks of land in settlement schemes, or taking over blocks when they became heads of household through death or divorce. In the World Bank report mentioned earlier, the authors observe that, while some change has occurred, 'it is still difficult for women to obtain permanent land management rights, and it is not uncommon to find that commercial land development decisions are made which ignore their gardening rights' (Brouwer *et al.* 1998, 10).

The low status of women and endemic violence against them have enormous implications for women's ability to avoid contracting HIV, for women confronting a positive HIV test result, and for women faced with the task of ensuring family survival while looking after a sick husband. As recently as last year, a case was reported of a group of young men who had attempted to seek compensation from the village court when it transpired that a woman they had raped was HIV-positive at the time of the rape.[4] Health-education messages promoting safer sex under these circumstances can ring hollow.

What is needed are models of development that can demonstrate a synergy between improvements in the status of women, and positive programme outcomes in relation to HIV. Without evidence of this nature, advocacy to promote gender equity often falls on deaf ears in PNG. In the following section, we move on to focus on the Mama Lus Frut Scheme, which we argue can show just such a synergy.

The Mama Lus Frut Scheme[5]

The oil-palm industry is one of the more successful industries in PNG. The industry leaders are, however, well aware of the importance to the industry of the smallholders who control 45 per cent of the planted area, and account for 25 per cent of the production.[6] The Oil Palm Industry Corporation (OPIC), part of the private sector in PNG, is constantly looking for ways to improve production by ensuring the maximum return from harvests. Eight years ago the Mama Lus Frut Scheme was introduced. The scheme was set up as part of an effort to improve oil-palm production by improving the collection of oil-palm fruit. Harvesters were being paid only for fruit harvested by the bunch.[7] Loose fruit, which fell from the bunches of oil palm before and during harvest, was being wasted.

Before the introduction of the scheme, all the money from harvesting bunches of fruit went to the smallholder, usually a man, who would then pay other, usually male, workers who had helped. Women only helped at harvest time, for payment; this was the case for a very small number of women. Smallholder production was recorded on a primary payment card, which was held by the male head of the smallholding. Wives, the majority of whom were not involved in harvesting, had less claim on the income from oil palm than those (mostly men) who had, so they would have to ask for cash to buy household necessities that they could not afford from the small income they got from selling garden produce, and other income-generating enterprises. The process of asking for cash was a constant source of acrimony between couples, leading to arguments and beatings.

The Mama Lus Frut Scheme specifically targeted women to collect the loose fruit that falls to the ground as the fruit bunches ripen. Women put this fruit in a separate pile next to the harvested bunches. This was seen as both improving efficiency by ensuring that the loose fruit was collected, and as enhancing the possibilities of greater economic independence for women. In the beginning, the scheme was seen purely as a way to increase production, and it was hoped by the designers of the scheme that 25 per cent of the income would go to women, which was proved correct as this stabilised quickly at about 26 to 27 per cent. As the scheme became established, OPIC realised that a spin-off of the scheme was the potential to reduce family conflicts among and within smallholder households. Other programmes focusing on economic empowerment for women and reporting similar results include the Intervention with Microfinance for AIDS and Gender Equity (IMAGE) in South Africa (Hargreaves *et al.* 2002) and the Shakti Sex Worker Projects in India and Bangladesh (UNAIDS 2000).

Under the scheme, cards continue to be used to register the number of bunches of fruit harvested from the block (the lorry that collects the fruit from the blocks 'clocks' the number collected at the time of pick-up). In addition to the card used to register men's harvesting, the Mama Lus Frut Scheme introduced a red 'Mama' card. The Mama pile is clocked by the collection lorry against the red card and the money transferred to the wife (or one of the women on the block, given that a block often accommodates several nuclear families).

Soon after the scheme was introduced, it was found that the male smallholders had begun to augment the Mama pile with a few bunches of harvested fruit to add to the income from that pile. It seems that the transfer of a few bunches of fruit to the Mama pile is a much more acceptable way for men to contribute to housekeeping funds than handing over cash to women (Koczberski *et al.* 2001, 181). The oil-palm milling company was resistant to the transfer of large quantities of whole fruit to the Mama pile, because deductions were made for loan repayments from the Papa card, not the

Mama card. This changed when debts began to be recovered firstly from the Papa card and then the Mama card if the agreed amount had not been reached, allowing modest transfers to take place once more (*ibid.*, 184). The amount earned per harvest varies, but a smallholder can expect to earn something in the region of 5,500 kina a year from oil palm (equivalent to £1,043 in August 2005). Twenty per cent of this is earned from the loose fruit, and is therefore allocated to the Mama card, with pay going directly to women.

The scheme was not intended as an HIV-focused intervention, but emerging evidence suggests that it may play an important role in the HIV response. This is because of its role in enhancing women's bargaining position within the household, increasing their voice. Evaluations of the scheme show that in the first years of operation the scheme has reduced conflict and domestic violence, as well as increased production overall, while providing a more equitable dispersal of benefits (Koczberski *et al.* 2001; Warner and Bauer 2002). Koczberski *et al.* (175) observe: 'For women, greater access to cash was welcomed, but it was the fact that they had more control over the income and hence less financial reliance on their husbands that was most important.' The benefits of the Mama Lus Frut Scheme mirror those of the IMAGE project in South Africa. IMAGE emphasises the importance of the environment in which sexual behaviours, gender-based violence, and HIV infections are occurring. In supporting disadvantaged women and households to be economically independent through micro-finance schemes, and strengthening community networks through participatory learning and action approaches,[8] IMAGE seeks to 'strengthen individual client agency and to improve household well-being, communication and power relations...[and]...has the potential to influence levels of gender-based violence and vulnerability to HIV/AIDS' (Hargreaves *et al.* 2002, 9).

The Mama Lus Frut Scheme may not have been intended to provide a way of enhancing women's position in the home in order to help prevent the spread of HIV, but with the growing threat that HIV poses to such a labour-intensive industry (International Finance Corporation 2002, 7), a scheme that has become 'core business' for the oil-palm industry is already likely to be playing a part in slowing the spread of HIV.

A new scheme has recently been piloted that introduces a third type of card – the 'mobile' card (Page 2004). This card will allow people who are short of labour, perhaps because of sickness, age, or simply a lack of people available during a particular harvest time, to engage young people, or members of their own *wantok* (extended family/friends who share the same language) to do the harvesting for them. The mobile card will allow these mobile workers to benefit from a part of the harvest. This scheme can cater not only for the needs of under-employed youth and other workers, but may potentially help people living with HIV and AIDS when sickness or death robs a smallholder of household and family members who would have provided labour. The adoption of this scheme requires changes to the software used for clocking harvests against payment cards and a higher level of management, so it is yet to be adopted on a large scale.

Thus, the Mama Lus Frut Scheme and the Mobile Card Scheme, which were both intended to increase oil-palm production and to address inequality in benefit sharing, may also provide avenues for arresting the spread of HIV and mitigating the impact of the epidemic. Improved social relations in general, and greater economic independence of women in particular, are key elements in a successful response to the HIV and AIDS epidemic in PNG and elsewhere. What is needed now is greater attention to the documentation of such initiatives, and the development of methods to measure the impact that such programmes have had on community perceptions and practices with regard to HIV.

For example, in the case of the Mama Lus Frut Scheme, has this enabled women to take more control of their sexuality? In terms of care, does the scheme enable greater social coherence, so that if someone is sick, others can support them? And are mobile cards likely to be used to assist HIV-affected households? At the moment, there are no answers to these questions. The potential impact of the Mama Lus Frut Scheme and the Mobile Card Scheme on people affected by HIV is unknown. It is hoped that these schemes, which aim to improve law and order, gender and family relations, and consequently improve production among oil-palm producers, also have potential benefits for reducing HIV transmission, given the intimate link between gender inequities, violence, drunkenness, and the spread of HIV. A thorough gender analysis of the impact of the schemes on intra-household relations is needed to ascertain if the hoped-for benefits outlined in this chapter are being realised, and to assess the potential for arresting the spread of HIV. There is a strong commitment in both OPIC and OPRA (the Oil Palm Research Agency) to addressing HIV and AIDS in the industry. Efforts are already being made to ensure that prevention messages are shared through the extension service.[9] There is also an awareness of the need for research on the gendered impact of the schemes described above; when this research is undertaken the findings will have the potential to inform interventions beyond the oil-palm industry, and beyond PNG.

Conclusion

Mainstreaming gender equity through a social model of development may have a significant impact on the HIV epidemic, because, even though addressing the epidemic is not the original purpose, schemes like those discussed in this chapter focus on the inequitable gender relations that play an important part in the spread of HIV. Ideally, in the near future the Mama Lus Frut and Mobile Card Schemes might be augmented, for example providing information on HIV, voluntary counselling and testing, condoms, and anti-retroviral therapy. The Mama Lus Frut Scheme provides an example of how mainstreaming HIV could be approached via livelihoods and economic development planners infusing their work with gender analysis, gender-sensitive research, and gender-equality goals.

This article was originally published in Gender & Development, *volume 14, number 1, March 2006.*

References

Asian Development Bank (2002) *Priorities of the Poor in Papua New Guinea*, Manila: ADB.

Association for Women's Rights in Development (2004) *Gender Mainstreaming: Can it Work for Women's Rights?*, Spotlight 3, November, Toronto, Canada: AWID.

Brouwer, E. C., B. M. Harris, and S. Tanaka (1998) *Gender Analysis in Papua New Guinea*, Washington DC: The World Bank.

Butcher, K. (2003) 'Lessons Learned from Mainstreaming HIV into the Poverty Eradication Action Plan in Uganda', report for DFID Uganda, London: John Snow International Research and Training UK, www.synergyaids.com/documents/Uganda_lessLearned_HIVPoverty.pdf (last accessed August 2007).

Dugue, M. (2004) 'PNG: a man's world?', *ADB Review* (January–February 2004), www.adb.org/Documents/Periodicals/ADB_Review/2004/vol36_1/world.asp (last accessed August 2007).

Government of PNG (2004) *Medium Term Development Strategy 2005–2010*, November 2004, Port Moresby: Department of National Planning and Rural Development, www.undp. org.pg/documents/mtds2005-10.pdf (last accessed August 2007).

Gustafsson, B. (2002) *Rural Households and Resource Management in Papua New Guinea*, RMAP Working Paper 32, Canberra: Resource Management in Asia-Pacific Program, The Australian National University.

Hargreaves, J., T. Atsbeha, J. Gear, J. Kim, B. M. Makhubele, K. Mashaba, L. Morison, M. Motsei, C. Peters, J. Porter, P. Pronyk, and C. Watts (2002) *Social Interventions for HIV/AIDS. Intervention with Micro-Finance for AIDS and Gender Equity*, IMAGE Study Evaluation Monograph No. 1, Acornhoek, South Africa: Rural AIDS and Development Action Research Programme.

International Finance Corporation (2002) *HIV in the Workplace*, Good Practice Note No. 2, December 2002, Washington DC: IFC.

Koczberski, G., G. N. Curry, and K. Gibson (2001) *Improving Productivity of the Smallholder Oil Palm Sector in Papua New Guinea*, Canberra: RSPAS, The Australian National University.

Lonely Planet (2005) '*Papua New Guinea*', www.lonelyplanet.com/worldguide/destinations/pacific/papua-new-guinea/ (last accessed November 2005).

Mgone, C. S., M. E. Passey, J. Anang, W. Peter, T. Lupiwa, D. M. Russell, D. Babona, and M. P. Alpers (2002) 'Human immunodeficiency virus and other sexually transmitted infections among female sex workers in two major cities in Papua New Guinea', *Sexually Transmitted Diseases* 29(5): 265–70.

National AIDS Council (2004) 'National Consensus Workshop Report', mimeo.

Newlin, A. (2000) 'The Effects of Economic Growth on Gender Roles in Papua New Guinea and the Tolai People', www.calibercreations.com/pisin/PNGstudy.htm (last accessed August 2007).

Page, W. (2004) 'A mobile income benefits everyone', *Partners in Research and Development*, December 2004: 4–5.

Passey, M., C. S. Mgone, S. Lupiwa, N. Save, S. Tiwara, T. Lupiwa, A. Clegg, and M. P. Alpers (1998) 'Community based study of sexually transmitted diseases in rural women in the highlands of Papua New Guinea: prevalence and risk factors', *Sexually Transmitted Infections* 74(2): 120–7.

UNAIDS (2000) 'Female Sex Worker HIV Prevention Projects: Lessons Learnt from Papua New Guinea, India and Bangladesh, UNAIDS Case Study', Geneva: UNAIDS.

UNAIDS (2004) *Facing the Future Together: Report of the Secretary-General's Task Force on Women, Girls and HIV/AIDS in Southern Africa*, Geneva: UNAIDS.

UNAIDS/UNICEF/WHO (2004) 'Papua New Guinea', Epidemiological Fact Sheets on HIV/AIDS and Sexually Transmitted Infections, Geneva: UNAIDS, www.who.int/hiv/pub/epidemiology/pubfacts/en/ (last accessed August 2007).

Warner, R. and M. Bauer (2002) *Mama Lus Frut Scheme: An Assessment of Poverty Reduction*, Impact Assessment Series No. 20, Canberra: ACIAR.

Windybank, S. and M. Manning (2003) *Papua New Guinea on the Brink*, Issue Analysis 30, St. Leonards, NSW, Australia: Centre for Independent Studies, www.cis.org.au/IssueAnalysis/ia30/ia30.htm (last accessed August 2007).

World Bank (2004) *Papua New Guinea: Poverty Assessment*, Washington DC: The World Bank.

Yawa, M. (n.d.) 'Gender and Violence', Royal Papua New Guinea Constabulary, www.aic.gov.au/conferences/policewomen3/yawa.pdf (last accessed August 2007).

Notes

1 Development workers in more than one country have told us this when we have opened discussion on HIV mainstreaming.

2 We take as our definition of gender mainstreaming 'a strategy which aims to bring about gender equality and advance women's rights by infusing gender analysis, gender-sensitive research, women's perspectives and gender equality goals into mainstream policies, projects and institutions' (Association for Women's Rights in Development 2004, 1).

3 Report in the *The Nation* (newspaper) on 12 May 2004 on the proceedings of the National Consensus Report Workshop, Port Moresby.

4 Personal communication with the Family and Sexual Violence Committee, pngfvac@daltron.com.pg.

5 We are very grateful to Frank Lewis (OPIC) for his comments and advice on this section.

6 An overview of the socio-economic aspects of the oil-palm industry can be found in a summary of research carried out by the Research Unit for the Study of Societies in Change, Curtin University of Technology, which is available at: http://research.humanities.curtin.edu.au/rus_research.cfm (last accessed August 2007).

7 The oil-palm fruits, which are the shape of tiny coconuts, cluster on a bunch shaped like a huge blackberry that hangs from the crown of the palm, with hundreds of individual fruits making up a single bunch.

8 More information on IMAGE can be found at: www.sarpn.org.za/mitigation_of_HIV_AIDS/m0025/index.php (last accessed August 2007).

9 Posters have been designed that show the potential impact of HIV on a smallholder family. These posters will be disseminated through the extension services, which are in very regular contact with all smallholders.

Part IV
Positive agency and action

12 Advocacy training by the International Community of Women Living with HIV/AIDS

The International Community of Women Living with HIV/AIDS

The International Community of Women Living with HIV/AIDS (ICW) is the only international network of HIV-positive women. Our members, in 134 countries, work with local, national, and international networks, organisations, and groups supporting and campaigning for the rights of HIV-positive women and men.

ICW was established in 1992 in response to the desperate lack of support, information, and services available worldwide to women living with HIV, and to enable these women to influence and contribute to official policy development. HIV-positive women from around the world attended the eighth International Conference on AIDS, held in Amsterdam in July 1992, where they shared stories and strategies for coping. They also devised action plans for the future. Because they did not want to lose the momentum created at the conference, ICW came into being. Our vision for ourselves and for all HIV-positive women is to create a world in which:

- we are involved in a respected and meaningful way in decision-making that affects our lives, at all political levels;

- we have access to full care and treatment, regardless of our age or lifestyle;

- all our economic, social, and political rights are respected, including our right to make choices concerning our sexual and reproductive lives, and our right to live free of discrimination in all areas of our lives, irrespective of our culture, age, religion, sexuality, social or economic status or class, and race.

At ICW, we believe that the second and third aspects of this vision will not be realised in the absence of the first. This is why ICW members around the world can be found advocating not merely for involvement, but for meaningful involvement, in decisions that affect our lives. Sadly, legal and policy changes are too often determined by people who do not understand the realities in which HIV-positive women live their lives. Our members know what it is to live with HIV, and they know what they need in order to improve their well-being, yet others continue to speak on our behalf or judge us. For women and men living with HIV and AIDS, meaningful participation in policy making and reporting on the impact of existing policies continues to be the exception rather than the rule. When it does occur, it tends to be tokenistic. We feel that, without greater – and better-integrated – political participation by HIV-positive women, we will not achieve the support that we need. As long as we are not the ones determining the direction of policies and programmes, genuine and positive change is unlikely to happen.

Factors that prevent women's participation in decision-making

In this section, I discuss some factors which limit the involvement of HIV-positive women in decision-making processes.

Negative attitudes

The following quotations illustrate the exclusion of HIV-positive women from forums where policies and decisions are made. (Like all quotations presented in this article, these come from workshops conducted in 2005 by ICW in Lesotho, Swaziland, and South Africa as part of a wider advocacy-focused project.)

- 'We are always submissive and do not challenge those in authority.'
- 'When you voice your idea, your idea is not accepted because of your status.'
- 'Our input is not implemented, and our ideas are not taken into consideration.'
- 'Men that are decision makers feel that women's place is in the kitchen. We don't feel part of the decision-making community.'
- 'We have organisations, but men lead them, and our issues don't get discussed.'
- 'Policymakers sit in board rooms and decide what is relevant to our lives – we are not part of the process.'

The marginalisation of HIV-positive women is not only a feature of main-stream policy arenas. National and international HIV organisations and networks should be a source of support for HIV-positive women, and should involve them fully in decision-making. However, they often reflect the gender discrimination that is found in society more generally. Despite women's strong presence in support groups, national (and international) groups of people living with HIV/AIDS are dominated by men. 'There is always a male AIDS activist responding to programmes on the TV and radio about HIV-positive women and pregnancy. An AIDS activist on the radio was asked about HIV-positive women having babies. He doesn't feel it is their right, yet he has two children' (ICW Rapid Assessment, South Africa 2005).

Practical issues

HIV-positive women are often overburdened with caring for others and bringing up children, as well as looking after their own health. Our members report that care and support for people infected or affected by HIV and AIDS is carried out almost exclusively by people (especially women) who are themselves infected or affected. Positive women are active in health-care settings, as counsellors, in home-based care, and in community education through churches, schools, and other community groups; they are often very active in setting up and administering support groups, and in providing for orphans and other vulnerable children, and for elderly people. Nearly all such work is done on a voluntary basis, without strong external support or official recognition, despite the fact that it is effectively supplementing the inadequate services that are available from governments and NGOs. Governments worldwide fail to provide the level of service that is required by people living with HIV and AIDS.

Alliances could be built between carers and service providers (actual and potential), and carers could be consulted about future policy and programming. There is plenty happening at the community level that could be used to influence policy or programme formulation, but no one is asking women 'What is the right thing to do?'. Furthermore, women living with HIV and AIDS are so busy providing community-level care and supporting service-delivery activities that they lack time and resources to apply their skills to other areas of involvement, such as advocacy, research, or leadership and co-ordination.

It seems that, although care and support work is important, it does not reach the attention of decision makers at the policy level because it is done on a voluntary basis. Yet it conveniently fills a gap in service provision which otherwise government policy makers would have to fill.

Lack of specific skills and knowledge

Those in power often tend to use women's lack of skills – actual, as a result of gender bias in education, training, or employment; or perceived, as an outcome of prejudice – as an excuse not to involve them in policy formulation or impact assessment. They commonly fail to recognise women's expertise and skills, and they do not attempt to support women to develop other skills through capacity-building programmes.

One of the reasons identified by ICW members for their lack of meaningful involvement was their lack of skills. 'People in government ask us, "can you formulate policies?", and we can't; we don't know where to start, how to approach people, and what questions to ask' (ICW workshop, Swaziland, 2005). Participants complained that when 'experts' (for example, those who determine HIV policy and programmes) had asked them, 'Do you have the skills to change policies?' and they said no, they were not taken seriously (*ibid.*).

Capacity-building needs to be a two-way process, in which governments and businesses and organisations learn how to encourage and facilitate the meaningful involvement of women carers. One participant in our workshops commented: 'People think asking positive women to come and speak is enough. They need to be educated' (*ibid.*). ICW believes that those in positions of power urgently need to build their own capacity – the capacity to engage with HIV-positive people in ways that are equitable, respectful, and productive for all involved.

Having raised some of the issues and identified the problems, in the next section I discuss some of the activities undertaken by ICW to break the deadlock.

Building bridges, confidence, and skills

At ICW, we have learned that developing advocacy skills and agendas cannot be done in a vacuum. Solidarity and support networks are vital prerequisites. ICW supports training workshops, and other programmes that are designed to do the following:

- expand outreach and create self-help groups, to reduce feelings of isolation and hopelessness;
- increase the self-esteem of HIV-positive women;
- increase individual skills that strengthen networks, which will result in a wider pool of supported, knowledgeable, and effective women advocates;
- train HIV-positive women to influence public opinion, policies, and service delivery at local and national levels. This will enhance services and reduce discrimination and stigma.

ICW has been facilitating exercises that help participants to identify what needs to change in government and NGO programmes, and how and where those changes should take place. These workshops have several particularly interesting features. They are context-specific, in that they focus on the lived experience of women in a specific geographical, political, and social context; they introduce or apply gender analysis to that context; they have as an end-point an advocacy message, agenda, plan, or tool, developed by, and for use by, the participants of the workshop; and they build the capacity of workshop participants to mobilise other members of their community to engage in similar activism.

The statements by HIV-positive women quoted earlier in this article were made during an ongoing project that has used this methodology to develop an advocacy-skills and advocacy-action plan in Swaziland and South Africa. This is described in the next section.

Advocacy training and development project: Swaziland and South Africa

ICW has joined forces with the POLICY project[1] and 40 HIV-positive women from Swaziland and South Africa. The agenda that has been developed focuses on asserting women's sexual and reproductive-health rights, and the right to full access to care, treatment, and support for women living with HIV/AIDS. The advocacy targets are being determined by the participants.

The project began with an assessment of the concerns and experiences of HIV-positive women in Swaziland and South Africa, and the policy and institutional environment in both countries. Information from the workshops was augmented by research and training conducted by ICW and POLICY with HIV-positive women in Swaziland.[2] This included a focus on women's access to treatment. In South Africa there has been little documentation of the experiences of HIV-positive women, so we conducted a further situation assessment with 21 women from rural and urban areas. Through this, we aimed to find out their experience within families, communities, health centres, support groups, and decision-making circles.

Women's decision-making power in sexual relationships

Women's assessment of their degrees of power in sexual relationships tended to vary, but generally they felt that they had less power than their male sexual partners to determine when and how to have sex. Comments included the following:

- 'Our partners use sex to own us.'
- 'They force us to have sex even if we don't want to.'
- 'They threaten to leave, or sleep with other women. If you refuse, the mood of the house becomes intense.'
- 'He does not force me to have sex, but he does emotionally, because if I don't, then I don't get money, he might leave or won't talk to me.'
- 'I am able to ask him to use a condom, but sometimes he refuses. That is why I stick to Femidom.'
- 'We use a male condom. It is because of our situation as a discordant couple,[3] and he never refuses.'

Caring for others when you need care yourself

Women talked of carrying the burden of caring for themselves and others: 'I was ill, and had to wake up and wash those nappies. I didn't have the strength.' … 'We have so many challenges, and no one to take care of our health. No one to say "take your nevarapine now".'

Community and family pressures

There was much discussion of community and family pressures on matters related to motherhood, sexuality, and sexual relations. Participants reported that family members often fail to support women's efforts to claim their sexual rights and reproductive rights. For example, in rural areas, wife inheritance is a big problem. One woman reported: 'Parents and in-laws get together to decide; the woman isn't part of the meeting, especially where *lobola* (bride-price) is paid, you are property.'

Another said: 'My brother-in-law wanted to take my husband's place. He didn't want to marry [me, but] he wanted a sexual relationship. [He said:] "If you don't do this, we won't support the child." I told him,"Get out" .'

Disclosing one's HIV status in a difficult environment

Women agreed that theirs is a particularly difficult environment in which to disclose their status. They fear blame, violence, and abandonment. Among the women at the workshop, disclosure had occurred gradually – it was not a one-off action after a single decision. Disclosure to partners, families, friends, neighbours in the surrounding communities, and the public in general involved differing degrees of anxiety, and problems that did not necessarily diminish with time. Stigma, discrimination, and lack of support from others are common reactions when women disclose their HIV status. One commented: 'If we disclose up-front, these guys won't want to be involved. If we disclose in the middle of a relationship, we might have to start another relationship.'

Lack of solidarity among women

Lack of solidarity among women was discussed. Most of the women felt comfortable discussing their issues with other HIV-positive women, but a number of them felt that women from beyond this group were not always supportive of them. There was lack of trust between women who were divided by other personal characteristics, including age, sexuality, socio-economic status, race, religion, and ability, and between rural and urban women. 'Women are divided – they are suspicious of each other', said one.

Lack of information

Lack of appropriate information for HIV-positive women on sexual and reproductive health, treatment and care, and nutrition was a concern for all: 'The information you get in health centres is government information. The basis is their programmes, so it is not necessarily on reproductive rights because that's not their stance – their stance is on how you should eat garlic.' ... 'There is information, but it is not independent from people that are selling the [medical] products – so it is not neutral.'

Information provided by NGOs was appreciated, but there were complaints that it is not always comprehensive enough to cover the needs of HIV-positive women, in that it tends to focus mainly on prevention.

Lack of full and appropriate health care

Women talked of the lack of appropriate, good-quality services for HIV-positive women, and the lack of cohesion between services. Family-planning advice, ante-natal services, treatment for sexually transmitted infections, and voluntary counselling and testing are offered in many but not all clinics and hospitals. This is especially the case in rural areas. Certain services are not always offered at the women's local or regular clinics.

Nearly all the women regretted the lack of services adapted to the needs and concerns of an HIV-positive woman. One woman commented: 'When I enter a clinic, I want to enter a woman's health centre where they know what to do.' In fact, opportunities to provide comprehensive care, treatment, and support are often missed. 'Service providers lack knowledge of proper treatment.' ... 'When you are stressed, herpes occurs – they tell you use a condom and they don't know it's not just when you have sex.'

There are widespread complaints about the judgemental attitudes of health-care service providers and their failure to respect confidences. Indeed, bad treatment by health-care workers was cited by the majority of women as a reason why they did not feel comfortable using official services. 'There is no confidentiality, privacy or dignity when you go to government clinics. Wherever you are, you get treated like an alien from Mars.'

Coercion and lack of choice in reproductive-health services, testing, and treatment uptake is another major issue. One woman said: '[If you are pregnant], they do not tell you, "if you keep it, a, b, or c is there for you" – they don't give you the option. They sterilise you. You feel obliged to take the option they offer you, or you feel you can't take the immediate service you need.'

The participants also reported not being given preparatory and follow-up tests when seeking anti-retroviral drugs (ARVs). Hence, they were not always given the correct combination and dosage at the right time. Some women felt pressured to take ARVs when they did not feel ready. '[The] problem goes beyond drugs – those on treatment should say that it is not just about ART, but about other treatments too. Care and support are important too.'

Lack of meaningful involvement in policy and programme formulation

Women discussed their lack of meaningful involvement when policies and programmes were being formulated. They resented the fact that others would speak on their behalf. 'We have organisations, but men lead the organisations, and our issues don't get discussed.'

Lack of involvement in research into prevention and treatment

It was generally felt by the women in the discussion workshops that research totally overlooked their priorities. For example, women needed microbicides, which prevent HIV transmission between sexual partners but permit women to become pregnant: 'They always focus on prevention and transmission, but what about HIV-positive people that want babies?

They don't bring HIV-positive women to be part of the research and to say what we think about their projects, instead of deciding for us.'

We found that there was a great deal of overlap between the experiences of the HIV-positive women from Swaziland and those of the women from South Africa. In relation to the quality of health care on offer, Swazi participants particularly complained that treatment was often not explained properly, a fact which drives away women who are seeking treatment. They reported being obliged to seek medication 'over the counter' from unqualified shop-keepers, or from traditional healers. In this situation, there is likely to be no monitoring and/or no follow-up. The participants emphasised the importance of informing women about treatment and where to get it, about the medication they have been prescribed, the likely side effects, and the expected benefits.

Consolidating and prioritising the issues for advocacy

Twenty women from Swaziland and the 20 women involved in the South African assessment met in Durban in June 2005 to discuss and prioritise the issues raised in the research phase of the project. They identified the following priorities that needed to be addressed: stigma and discrimination; disclosure of HIV status; the need for access to proper care, treatment, and support; and the need for improved information on sexual and reproductive health and rights. In addition, two related areas that received particular attention were HIV testing and the criminalisation of people living with HIV and AIDS.

Testing

Currently the focus on HIV testing in many countries throughout the world, including South Africa and Swaziland, is on ante-natal testing. Although participants recognised the importance of testing pregnant women, they felt that the almost exclusive focus on testing women at ante-natal clinics meant that women were discovering their status at a very stressful time of their lives, and risked being perceived as bringing HIV into the family. Although participants welcomed more flexible opportunities for testing, they were also extremely concerned about plans to scale-up testing and to introduce a policy of routine testing.

Scaling-up testing is a cause for worry when current testing practices do not always ensure informed and voluntary consent. Some women at the workshop had heard about women being tested without any proper explanation of what they were being tested for, or even knowing whether or not they had been tested for HIV. 'I know an HIV-positive woman who was told to get tested, but she knew nothing, and then she was told she was positive. They gave her the meds without details, and she uses some meds for her kids because she does not understand.'

Where testing is routine and supposedly voluntary, women and men may not be aware that they have the right to opt out. However, asserting that women can opt out is meaningless in a context where there is an unequal power relationship between service providers and service users. When service providers recommend women to take a test, the women often comply because the service providers are in a position of authority, and the clients may not realise that they can choose to say no. When women go home, they face pressures from family and communities concerning their sexual and reproductive lives. These may result in stigmatisation, violence, and abandonment.

Criminalisation

In South Africa, wilful transmission of HIV is a criminal offence (whether the perpetrator is a man or a woman). It is regarded as a sexual offence equivalent to rape. The women at the workshop felt strongly that HIV-negative people should bear the responsibility for protecting their own sexual health; but they also recognised that many women, particularly younger women, were not in such a position. 'Criminalisation is hard to enforce, because how do we know if a person was aware of their status? It's a law that could protect women, but where do we draw the line of confidentiality?' Criminalisation may put pressure on people to disclose their positive status before they feel ready to do so, with consequences that might include violence, abuse, loss of livelihoods, and abandonment. Conversely, it may discourage people from getting tested.

Training and advocacy planning

The actual training and advocacy planning took place over five days in August 2005, with the same 40 women. We discussed the steps involved in advocacy, considering examples of participants' own experiences of using advocacy opportunities to achieve change in the two countries. The training workshop combined background knowledge, sharing of experiences, skills development, and planning, with the objective of producing a number of advocacy action plans that could be implemented in the coming months with continued support from ICW and POLICY Project.

The policy and institutional environment

Analysing the policy and institutional environment in both countries was vital in order to ensure that participants understood the opportunities for advocacy and the constraints that compromised the chances of success.

Both Swaziland and South Africa have signed agreements that should protect the sexual and reproductive rights of HIV-positive women. These include the Convention on the Elimination of All Forms of Discrimination Against Women (CEDAW), the United Nations International Conference on Population and Development (ICPD) Platform and Programme of Action

(1994), and the Windhoek Declaration (2005). This most recent agreement, signed by all the health ministers of the continent, focuses on upholding the sexual and reproductive rights of women in Africa.

Although these documents are not specific to HIV-positive women, we all share the same rights, and they can be used for leverage in advocacy initiatives. But unfortunately, the rights endorsed in these documents have yet to be reflected in national policies and programmes on HIV, AIDS, and sexually transmitted infections. Such programmes and policies continue to ignore the rights of HIV-positive women. This is no doubt a direct result of the women's lack of involvement in decision-making, as described above. Governments' lack of consideration for the rights of HIV-positive women was demonstrated all too harshly at our workshop: the government representative who had been invited to give a presentation (and who had confirmed an intention to attend) failed to attend the event, without bothering even to offer an excuse.

There is, however, some movement for change. Swaziland does have a draft policy on gender equality – although it has been in draft form since 2000. The Swazi government is also developing a policy and strategy on reproductive health, with input from POLICY and ICW. South Africa, on the other hand, is developing a bill on equity in marriage, and care and confidentiality in the health sector.

Although they are not sufficiently specific for HIV-positive women, these draft laws and policies do provide advocacy opportunities for our members. During the workshop we examined these policy documents. ICW had been invited by those drafting the policies to give feedback on them, with provision for participants' comments to be fed directly into current efforts to influence policy makers. For example, one of the articles in the Equity in Marriage Bill states that couples should be tested for HIV before they are married, and the women at the workshop were alarmed about the possible fate of a woman if she tested positive at this stage.

Examples of advocacy work

Some of the participants were invited to share examples of advocacy from their own personal experience, and this was used as a basis for identifying the various components of the advocacy process. Two examples of advocacy cited by our participants are included here.

On hearing that the Swazi army refused to recruit people living with HIV, one of the participants had tried to join up in order to raise people's awareness of this discrimination. She was paraded naked in front of a male doctor, then told she could not join because she had keloids (scar tissue), and her 'blood was bad'. The ICW Southern African Co-ordinator is working with women in Swaziland to try to get this discriminatory regulation overturned.

A number of activists in South Africa have recently formed a coalition called Womandla, which aims to ensure that the voices of HIV-positive women are heard in national responses to HIV. One of their first objectives was to attend a recent national AIDS conference in Durban. However, the registration fee was greater than the cost of six months' worth of anti-retroviral drug treatment. They picketed at the conference, and were eventually able to secure entry for three of their number.

Examples of advocacy work were also given by external presenters from the Treatment Action Campaign, the Reproductive Health Alliance, and Women In Law In Southern Africa (Swaziland). They helped us to understand advocacy strategies used by other organisations, and they formed part of an important and ongoing process of building alliances. This programme is supported by a reference group consisting of women from a number of key organisations working on women's rights and HIV, who offered their support in the development and implementation of advocacy strategies.

Developing advocacy plans

The following advocacy goals were chosen, and plans were developed accordingly.

Goal: To make available alternative technologies which prevent the transmission of HIV while allowing conception.

How? By demanding that government should incorporate appropriate measures into already existing family-planning programmes.

Goal: to guarantee the sexual and reproductive rights of HIV-positive women, including the right to good-quality services.

How? By urging the Ministry of Health to provide in all regional hospitals by 2010 annual pap smears for HIV-positive women, and free monitoring tests such as CD4 counts and viral load services, and breast-cancer services.

Goal: to involve HIV-positive women – in an ethical manner – in research.

How? Initially by promoting existing methodologies that effectively incorporate a gender-equality approach in academic institutions and among researchers.

Goal: To ensure that the rights of HIV-positive women in rural and urban areas are protected in their homes and communities.

How? By demanding the development of a policy that protects and enforces the property rights of all HIV-positive women (by December 2006).

Goal: to enable HIV-positive women to adopt children.

How? By calling on Swaziland's government to develop an adoption policy by December 2008 to allow HIV-positive women to adopt children freely.

Goal: Care and support for HIV-positive women in their communities.

How? By building the capacity of 200 HIV-positive women in their communities so that by June 2006 they have knowledge of the health services that are currently offered to 50 women in each region of Swaziland, through health centres and government hospitals.

We now have seven exciting advocacy action plans which the 40 participants, with support from ICW staff, will aim to implement over the coming months. There are many obstacles ahead, but with combined strength we hope to ensure better polices and programmes for HIV-positive women and their families and communities.

To conclude this article, one of the participants reflects on the workshop and the challenges facing HIV-positive women activists in implementing their plans:

'On my side a big gap was covered in the August workshop. Gaining skills was the main goal I wanted to achieve in this workshop. We were able to put down our action plans, which we hope will be implemented. I learned how to be an active advocate, how other people have advocated for something before. Knowing the outcomes of their actions helps to find an effective way of advocating. I learned how to put down strategies and smart objectives.

'We face a big problem when challenging our enemies. The problem might be that the person who is an enemy to us is the very person who is supposed to fall under our allies' list, e.g men are against condoms yet they should protect themselves, the next thing they blame a lady for bringing such disease at home. Another challenge is funding. It is very hard to get a kick start for funding. A further challenge at the time of writing in Swaziland is that it is impossible to find a complete policy document. Almost all the copies of policies that we have to use to inform our advocacy work are drafts, which makes it hard to implement. We also do not have individual champions who are HIV-positive women in high positions to help us push for the implementation.

'Another challenge is that people still believe that if you are HIV-positive you [are] suppose[d] to be sick or having opportunistic infections or... a sign which shows that you are positive. If a person like me is advocating for such issues, they just say that I am lying, I do that because I am given some money, meaning that I was bribed. For example, when I was exhibiting at the trade fair,[4] people would just come now and then, thinking that I will change my story. For example someone came twice and more, saying "Anya, come on now, the game is over, I would really like to know if you are a lady living with HIV or you just making a joke with it. I have been thinking about it overnight, you just want us to test, and what I can tell you is that you know nothing about issues for HIV-positive people, you don't know what they go through, so get a life". Man, it's surprising because these people are just like me. What I can say is that it takes an arm and a leg to be an advocate, but I am really proud of carrying out such work, as I know that not only allies will benefit from that but also enemies.'

This article was originally published in the name of Emma Bell in Gender & Development, *volume 13, number 3, November 2005.*

Notes

1 The POLICY Project endeavours to improve policies affecting family planning, reproductive health, HIV/AIDS, and maternal health programmes and services in developing countries. Multi-sectoral collaboration, community empowerment, respect for human rights and gender equality, and support for vulnerable populations, including orphans and other children affected by HIV/AIDS, characterise POLICY's approach to policy and programme development.

2 In October 2004, ICW ran an advocacy training workshop with 20 HIV-positive young women from Swaziland, and in February 2005 another workshop with 20 HIV-positive women, with the aim of monitoring government commitment to the rights of HIV-positive women. A similar workshop was held in Lesotho.

3 A 'discordant couple' is a couple in a sexual relationship in which one person is HIV-negative and the other is HIV-positive.

4 The trade fair is an event that occurs yearly in Swaziland in the summer. ICW has run a stand there, together with SWAPOL (Swaziland Positive Living).

Conclusion

Alice Welbourn

This collection has highlighted the immense global, psychosocial, economic, legal, and political issues facing us today in relation to the spread of HIV and AIDS. It has focused in particular on the gender dimension to this pandemic, the dimension which arguably is the one least recognised by the world's leaders. In this conclusion I seek to look beyond the issues covered in this collection, to touch on some of the other current and future challenges involved in responding to HIV and AIDS in an effective and gender-sensitive way. Of course, this conclusion cannot cover *every* challenge that has not been addressed in this book. There are many important issues that are not included here: the sex trade, international trafficking of girls and women, and the importance of keeping girls (both HIV-negative and HIV-positive) in school, for example.[1] Rather, what follows represents what I consider to be the most significant challenges for those working in this field.

Gender and the experiences of HIV-positive men

There is quite a large amount of literature on the gender dimensions of *why* men become HIV-positive. In most countries of the world, boys are brought up to be 'macho', and to have multiple sexual partners to demonstrate their dominance and virility. Men and boys are expected to know all about how their reproductive and sexual organs work, though few actually do. If they want to find information or health care related to sexual or reproductive health issues, such resources are scarce, even in the West. Violence, peer pressure, and lack of educational or economic opportunities exacerbate the vulnerabilities of young men to HIV, as shown in Chapters 3 and 7. In many countries, men and boys who are gay, bisexual, or questioning their sexual identity, keep their sexuality hidden, for fear of experiencing discrimination, homophobia, and related dominant behaviour or violence directed at them by other men intent on 'proving' their heterosexuality. This means they have even less access to important sex education, to condoms, or to relevant health care. All this is known. However, there is little literature to date on the *gender* dimensions of men's experiences, whatever their sexual orientation, once they are HIV-positive.

There are different reasons for this. Many men who identify as gay who are also HIV-positive do not connect their own experiences with the word 'gender', and prefer to talk about 'HIV and sexuality'. HIV-positive heterosexual men have not, on the whole, formed groups of mutual support or activism in the way that the male gay or female positive movement have.[2] The dominant – and false – belief in many countries that only 'gay' men can get HIV also deters many heterosexual men from disclosing their HIV status to others, again because of their own or others' homophobia. Yet globally, most men, from all levels of society, have acquired HIV through heterosexual sex. Even without homophobia, heterosexual men may still feel that they will be laughed at or scorned by others if they are found to be HIV-positive. This has meant that many heterosexual HIV-positive men become even more isolated and depressed than many of their gay or female counterparts. HIV-positive men who are or have been injecting drug users have added stigma to deal with because of attitudes towards drug use. HIV-positive men who acquired HIV through blood transmission because of haemophilia also have their own particular challenges related to physical and mental health, and economic stresses. Very little is known about HIV-positive transgendered men's – and women's – experiences, as Barbara Earth points out in Chapter 6.

GNP+, the only international network of HIV-positive people, has recently initiated a new programme focusing on the sexual and reproductive rights of men as well as women. It is hoped that this will do much to complement the long history of work by ICW on a gendered analysis of women's sexual and reproductive rights, and redress the paucity of research in this area. For instance, new research findings suggest that male circumcision provides some protection against HIV, but how can this information best be used while recognising that many circumcised men have still contracted HIV?[3]

Gender, HIV, and the global women's movement

In general, HIV-positive women and girls experience more stigma and discrimination than HIV-positive men and boys around the world (Paxton *et al.* 2004). This appears to be closely connected to the dominant belief in all societies that females are supposed to be the keepers of morality in society, and that an HIV-positive status is somehow immoral.[4] For HIV-positive women and girls, lack of support from most of the global women's movement for the past 25 years has been a particularly painful experience, and one which is not easy to explain. Thankfully, this is at last beginning to change, albeit slowly. One strong example of this is the leadership of the

World YWCA, a global network of 25 million women. The 2007 world council meeting, held in Nairobi, included at least one openly HIV-positive woman from each of the 100 country delegations, plus another 400 HIV-positive women out of a total meeting of 2,000 women. The whole conference, dedicated to HIV and AIDS, produced a wide-ranging ten-point personal call to action.[5] A historic leap forward indeed. It is hoped that other women's organisations will follow.

Education is not enough

While there is now clear evidence that access to school education for girls and young women can reduce risk from infection (UNAIDS 2006a; Hargreaves and Boler 2006), and may also reduce the impact of HIV infection, as Mushunje explains in Chapter 2, a school education alone is not enough to protect against HIV. In addition to schooling, well-designed, targeted gender-sensitive prevention strategies have the potential to help young people to protect themselves from infection. But to date, many prevention models have been criticised for their lack of gender awareness, and their lack of relevance to the everyday realities of young – or older – people. Much has been written, for instance, about the lack of gender sensitivity in the 'Abstain, Be faithful, use Condoms' (ABC) prevention model.[6] The more recent morality-driven abstinence-only and anti-condom campaigns favoured by the Bush regime have demolished much good prevention work in many countries.[7] These strategies are highly dangerous, as they only serve to give women in particular a false sense of security against the virus, misleading them into believing that they can protect themselves if they only have sex with one male partner. If they discover that they have become HIV-positive, such women often find themselves feeling ashamed and extremely shocked, because such simplistic prevention messages suggest that only the most stupid or immoral people, who surely only have themselves to blame, can get infected. Yet as many of the chapters in this volume have shown, such messages could not be further from the truth. Instead, it has become increasingly clear that good prevention education needs to include much broader gender-awareness training, and support for people of all genders to understand *why* we behave in the ways we do. Assertiveness training, communication and relationship skills, conflict resolution, economic independence, knowledge about how our bodies function, and knowledge about our rights are all also essential components of effective prevention education.

New technologies

In addition to the male condom, demonised both by the Bush regime and by the previous Pope (Jean Paul II),[8] other new technologies such as the female condom and microbicides offer hope to women and men as a form of prevention, and to prevent onward infection for HIV-positive people. A vaginal microbicide in particular offers new hope to HIV-positive women – and men – that they may be able to have children if they want to, while both protecting themselves from further exposure to HIV or other sexually transmitted infections (STIs), and protecting their partners from infection.[9] So far, though, with the exception of the biomedical research funded by the Gates Foundation, there has been no major investment either in female-condom production or in microbicide research, since these are seen by major companies as sideline 'women's issues' rather than mainstream initiatives (UNAIDS 2006b). In addition, microbicide development and female-condom promotion often just focus on HIV-negative people (see Welbourn 2006). Research should also focus on use by people with HIV and AIDS to prevent further transmission and to enable positive men and women to fulfil their rights to have sex, and to have children if that is what they want.

Ante-natal testing, sexual and reproductive rights, and access to care, treatment, and support

As discussed in Chapter 5 by Carolyn Baylies, for the most part, health institutions and public-health policies do not recognise sufficiently the key social, economic, and gendered dimensions to health, sickness, and health-care provision. This is in part because few health professionals at the national level, and in international institutions such as the World Health Organization, receive any gender training as part of their studies. And since inadequate research has been conducted in these areas, it is often easy for such issues to be dismissed, on the grounds that there is no evidence to show that gender is relevant to them.

For instance, it is now standard practice in many places to provide HIV testing to pregnant women when they attend ante-natal clinics. This provides a convenient opportunity to reach women. However, no matter how well-intentioned the idea of reaching out to women and protecting their children from infection, there is a strong sense from many activist quarters that women are yet again being seen first and foremost as objects, as reproductive vessels and 'disease vectors',[10] rather than as individuals in their own right. Now that most countries have adopted 'provider-initiated offer of testing' as routine, many pregnant women have found themselves saying yes to a test because they feel worried that if they say no they will be judged or maltreated – or not treated at all – by the health-care provider. Indeed, health-centre staff in many countries tell clients that the test is compulsory and that without it, no further care will be available for them (Anderson 2006). Many women, on receipt of a positive test result, are deeply shocked, and full of fear that they are about to die, and that their unborn child – and other children – may soon be motherless. They may also face violence from their partners and other family members, since it is often assumed that when a woman is the first to test positive in the family, she must surely be the one to have introduced HIV into the relationship. This is despite repeated insistence from many women in this situation that they are monogamous in their marriages and were virgins when they married.[11] There is an ever more pressing need for initiatives which promote voluntary couple counselling *before* conception[12] and, better still, which promote community-wide care and support and voluntary testing, on an opt-*in*, rather than an opt-*out* basis. In this way, the burden of knowledge of infection can be spread and shared across a fully supportive community, and the focus of blame on certain individuals – male, female, or transgender – can be eradicated (Bell *et al.* 2007).[13]

Similar gender issues arise in relation to international health-policy guidelines, donor funding, and national policies and practice in relation to care, treatment, and support.[14] Many of these policies undermine women's immense efforts to keep themselves alive, their families together, and to stop their children becoming orphans. This is because little attention has been paid by health-care planners or providers to the socio-economic or legal contexts of women's treatment, both within clinics and beyond the clinic door.[15] In many countries now, women outnumber men in attendance at public-health facilities in towns where anti-retroviral drugs are offered. However, research by ICW has shown that women often face problems with transport costs to reach the centres, child-care costs, and obtaining permission from family members to travel. Once at the clinic, they may face costs for related blood tests, compulsion to agree to long-term contraceptive injections or sterilisation before being given ARVs (thereby eroding their rights to motherhood – no equivalent conditions are demanded of men), and lack of access to condoms, cervical smears,[16] abortions, or drugs for other common STIs or co-infections, such as herpes, TB, hepatitis, or malaria.

Land, property, inheritance, and child custody

As White and Morton point out, property and custody issues relate to both the causes and effects of HIV from a gender perspective. Many women stay in relationships which they may realise are unsafe for them, for instance when they know that their husband is having unprotected sex with other partners, because they are fearful of what may happen to them if they leave the relationship. And some women also fear for the children they would have to leave behind, because in many societies, women hold no custody rights over their children. Many women, once they have nursed their sick husbands and become widows, find their land, homes, other property, and also their children taken away from them by the husband's family. This does not just happen in sub-Saharan Africa, as Kaori Izumi highlighted in her chapter on land-grabbing in the first volume of this series (on gender-based violence), but has also been reported widely by ICW members in the Asia-Pacific region and in Latin America. One HIV-positive woman in Latin America, who had started her own successful primary school, found that her dead husband's relatives spread the (false) rumour that she had infected him, thereby ensuring that parents removed their children from the school and the business collapsed. Her in-laws then seized the school building and contents from her and gave it to one of their relatives to run under new management.[17]

Drug use, gender, and HIV

The vulnerability to HIV and to hepatitis co-infection of all people who inject drugs is an area of huge and growing concern, particularly in South-East and South Asia, and Eastern Europe. In Myanmar, young male migrant labourers who work in the mines are 'paid' in morphine in order to dull the pain of the cold water in which they have to work. Elsewhere, many female drug users end up working in the sex industry against their will, often to pay for drugs for themselves and for their male partners, who may act as their pimps. Male, female, and transgender HIV-positive drug users are all likely to have contracted the infection in differing circumstances, and once infected, are likely to receive different care and support as a result of their gender identities (ICW 2007a). A particular issue faced by HIV-positive women who are or have been drug users is that they may be denied their rights to motherhood by judgemental health services, as well as being denied their rights to be involved in decisions which affect their lives.

Gender, research, and validation of knowledge

There is a hierarchy of knowledge associated with HIV. The medical dimension of the pandemic is at the top of this hierarchy. Formal scientific randomised control trials (RCTs)[18] are used as the gold standard of scientific evidence for interventions. However, such trials are very expensive, take several years, are considered by many to be unethical, and are not suited to understanding motivation and behaviour changes, or analysing feelings or emotions. Qualitative social science research methods, such as focus-group discussions and interviews with key informants, are considered by the medical community to be less robust than RCTs, and could be said to be second in the hierarchy of knowledge. But these methods often allow researchers to analyse complex human relationships and interactions, and often provide more understanding of what is happening to people.

At a third level there are participatory research methods, widely recognised as a valid way of recording the voices of women and men in communities involved in research projects.[19] They can also benefit from the agency of HIV-positive women and others at high risk as they analyse their own life experiences, and look at *why* what has happened to them has happened, suggesting changes in laws and practices which they consider will be most effective in ensuring that others do not face the same dilemmas. However, much of this participatory research, while remarkably uniform in its findings across continents, is regularly dismissed as 'anecdotal' and unscientific by the formal academic research, policy-making, and donor communities. As well as denying the legitimacy of an important source of knowledge about HIV and its impact, this is also a human-rights issue, since women – and HIV-positive women in particular – are normally least able to access the skills and resources required to carry out research using more formal methods. This means that they are constantly excluded from contributing to the accepted knowledge base which fuels policy and practice. To rectify this, ICW proposes that all NGOs, governments, UN agencies, donors, other development institutions, and the media engage with research and publications conducted by HIV-positive people, especially women, whose views are so often overlooked.

Lastly, there is still a huge lack of, and need for, sex- (and age-) disaggregated data in HIV and AIDS-related research. Where other health conditions have been studied, such as TB and malaria, gender disparities for diagnosis and treatment access are clearly seen (Silvester *et al.* 2005). Until such disagreggated data are more widely available in HIV and AIDS research, it would seem most appropriate for all policy makers, implementers, and donors to adopt the precautionary principle – i.e. to err on the side of caution and seek to 'do no harm' regarding the gender dimension to HIV interventions.[20]

Pharmaceutical companies and drug trials

Two key issues around pharmaceutical companies in relation to gender and HIV stand out. The first is a failure to include significant numbers of women in trials for new HIV drugs, which would produce more information about how HIV drugs might affect women's bodies. For instance, limited research has been carried out into how ARVs interact with the contraceptive pill and hence, whether it is safe for women to use both at the same time.[21] But more research is needed on this subject, and on the effects of ARVs on women's long-term fertility, or on the foetus, in order to allow HIV-positive women to make informed decisions about contraceptive use, and whether or not to try and get pregnant while taking ARVs. The second issue relates to overall pricing policies, drug licences, and blocks to the production of generic drugs. The removal of the latter in particular would bring ARV prices down, and make ARVs more available to women, who are often those least able to afford them.[22]

Promoting gender equity and HIV self-awareness in institutions

Globalisation has both spread the demand for luxury portable goods to new audiences in the South, and driven the production of cheap imports for the

North through promoting migrant labour in the South. Girls and boys are subject to immense peer pressure in many parts of the world to purchase consumer goods, from mobile phones to fashionable clothes; and for those who don't have their own means of buying them through their own incomes, transactional sex for girls (Weissman *et al.* 2006) and boys, and violent theft for boys (Walsh and Mitchell, this volume) are two very obvious alternatives. These activities, in turn, make girls and boys alike very vulnerable to HIV, through unprotected sex, gang rape, and exposed wounds. Concentrations of people involved in migrant labour, whether male or female, are also vulnerable to HIV, as Msimang highlights in this volume. There is thus an urgent and critical need for the commercial sector as a whole to address its part in the spread of HIV from a gendered perspective, in terms of the products it promotes and the means it uses to advertise them.

Many faith-based organisations also have much to do to reform their traditional attitudes towards men's and women's roles in society, and their attitudes towards people with HIV. Some faith groups are starting to make good progress, but these remain exceptions. Many faith-based organisations have done much to provide care and support for HIV-positive people. However, often these programmes reinforce traditional gender stereotypes by relying on volunteer, home-based care provided only by women who are often themselves HIV-positive (UNAIDS 2006c), while the paid project-management posts are still held by men.

NGOs, academic institutes, teacher-training institutes, government ministries, and the UN, are all heavily involved in the 'AIDS circus'.[23] They are also (with a very few rare exceptions) institutions heavily dominated by men in decision-making roles, many of whom have had no gender training, and have no political will or incentive to develop more gender-sensitive ways of working. They also contain many people with HIV, all struggling in their own lives with the issues discussed here.[24] Fundamental gender injustices form the foundations and fabric of all these institutions. These injustices need to be unpacked, dismantled, and redressed within the institutional structures first, if any of these institutions can hope to work effectively and in a sustainable way on gender and HIV.[25]

Within most institutions, there is certainly more public awareness of the human, emotional, and psychological dimensions to people's lives than there used to be. But most senior managers are still of a generation which has not been socially conditioned to address their own or others' psychological issues, nor to address homophobia, for instance, or the subordinate position of women, in their lives or in their work. And even women in senior positions often adopt 'masculine' methods of management, in order to survive in male-dominated working environments (Dickson 2003). These are not criticisms, just facts. So most development institutions are led by senior managers who are themselves ill-equipped to deal with the very issues which are now most deeply affecting their own staff – and possibly their own lives as well – and the members of the communities with whom those staff work.

Greater involvement of people with HIV and AIDS

Not surprisingly, one of the main consequences of an HIV diagnosis is clinical depression (WHO 2005). Yet many ICW members have described how getting involved in doing something to help others has actually helped them to manage better, psychologically, than those who don't or can't. So if any of you have reached the end of this volume and still doubt the importance of meaningfully involving women – and men – with HIV in your programme research, planning, implementation, monitoring or evaluation, then think about it as a good way to keep us living positively and productively. As development workers, we have a unique opportunity to build on all that we have learnt over the last 20 years about the importance of participatory practices, community-led initiatives, ownership and inclusion, in order to stem the tide of this pandemic. Yet the very people with whom we should be engaging most – those who are already HIV-positive – are often those who remain excluded and most stigmatised in the response to HIV to date. And at the bottom of this excluded pile you will repeatedly find HIV-positive women, who are so often doing the bulk of the voluntary caring work, but who are still rarely in key paid decision-making posts.[26] I hope that this collection has, if nothing else, encouraged you to think about ways of engaging men, women, and others with HIV, in a meaningful, positive, inclusive, and effective rights-based response to HIV and AIDS.

Positive futures

Gender injustices, violence, poverty, war, religious and racist hatred, and now HIV are insidious realities on all the continents of the world. Despite these, humans have continued to show the most extraordinary generosity, resilience, and compassion, as well as the ability to turn these negative forces into opportunities for positive change. As the powerful chapters in this volume have shown us, the reality of HIV challenges us to question and re-evaluate our values, assumptions, and deepest taboos, to banish hypocrisy and embrace the realities of our common human condition. Very few of us would have been born had our parents not had sex. If we now dare to accept that our sexuality (whether we have sex or not) is as much a part of the human condition as breath, water, food, and our universal inter-dependence, maybe we can all benefit in some way from this tragedy. Whoever and wherever we are in the world, we all seek happiness for ourselves and those we love, and we all wish to avoid suffering. Now could be the time for us at last to unite and call for a different way of running the world, a different way of relating to each other. We could create communities where sexual relations were based on consensual care, respect, pleasure, and safety, by mutual agreement between communicating adults, rather than on power, non-communication, violence, and oppression.

Patricia Perez, a Regional Representative of ICW Latina, who has been HIV-positive for 21 years, has just been nominated for the Nobel Peace Prize. If we humans, of whatever gender, are unable to find peace, liberty, safety, love, and respect in our own homes and communities, how can we ever hope to find peace in the wider world? Surely it follows that the solution to world peace and all its associations begins in our own homes and communities. Our universal response to the joint pandemics of HIV and AIDS, violence, and gender inequality is therefore critical for the futures of all of us. I for one certainly hope that Patricia wins that Nobel Prize. We all need this peace in our lives right now.

References

Anderson, B. (2006) 'A Human Rights Approach to HIV Testing: Voluntary, Mandatory or Routine?', Cape Town: AIDS Legal Network, available at: www.icw.org/files/ALQ%20Sept%202006%20-testing%20-.pdf (last accessed September 2007).

Bell, E., P. Mthembu, S. O'Sullivan, and K. Moody (2007) 'Sexual and reproductive health services and HIV testing: perspectives and experiences of women and men living with HIV and AIDS', *Reproductive Health Matters* 15 (29) 113–35, available at: www.icw.org/files/RHM29%20Suppl%20-%20Bell.pdf (last accessed September 2007).

Chirenje, Z. M., S. Rusakaniko, L. Kirumbi, E. W. Ngwalle, P. Makuta-Tlebere, S. Kaggwa, W. Mpanju-Shumbusho, and L. Makoae (2001) 'Situation analysis for cervical cancer diagnosis and treatment in East, Central and Southern African countries', *Bulletin of the World Health Organization* 79 (2): 127–32, available at: http://whqlibdoc.who.int/bulletin/2001/issue2/79(2)127-132.pdf (last accessed September 2007).

Dickson, A. (2003) *A Voice for Now: Changing the Way we See Ourselves as Women*, London: Piatkus Books.

Hargreaves, J. and T. Boler (2006) 'Girl power: the impact of girls' education on HIV and sexual behaviour', London: ActionAid, available at www.actionaid.org.uk/doc_lib/girl_power_2006.pdf (last accessed September 2007).

International Community of Women Living with HIV/AIDS (ICW) (2007a) 'HIV positive women and drug and alcohol use', ICW Vision Paper No. 6, London: ICW, available at: www.icw.org/files/24357%20English%20VP%206.pdf (last accessed September 2007).

International Community of Women Living with HIV/AIDS (ICW) (2007b) 'Global Call to stop cervical cancer', London: ICW, available at: www.icw.org/node/304 (last accessed September 2007).

Paxton, S., A. Welbourn, P. Kousalya, A. Yuvaraj, S. Pradhan Malla, and M. Seko (2004) '"Oh! This one is infected!": Women, HIV & Human Rights in the Asia-Pacific Region', paper presented at the Expert Meeting on HIV/AIDS in Asia-Pacific, Bangkok, 23–24 March 2004, available at: www.icw.org/files/ACJ0SB~2.PDF (last accessed September 2007).

Silvester, L., J. Raven, J. Price, S. Theobald, I. Makwiza, S. Jones, N. Kilonzo, R. Tolhurst, M. Taegtmeyer, and G. Dockery (2005) 'Analysis of the gender dimension in the scale-up of antiretroviral therapy and the extent to which free treatment at point of delivery ensures equitable access for women', Liverpool: Gender and Health Group, Liverpool School of Tropical Medicine, Liverpool Associates in Tropical Health; Nairobi: Liverpool VCT, Care & Treatment; Lilongwe: Reach Trust, available at: www.liv.ac.uk/lstm/research/groups/documents/report_gender_equity _art_scale_up.pdf (last accessed September 2007).

UNAIDS (2006a) 'Educate girls, fight AIDS', Geneva and Washington DC: UNAIDS, available at: http://data.unaids.org/GCWA/GCWA_FS_ GirlsEducation_Sep05_en.pdf (last accessed September 2007).

UNAIDS (2006b) 'Increase women's control over HIV prevention, fight AIDS', Geneva and Washington DC: UNAIDS, available at: http://data.unaids.org/ pub/BriefingNote/2006/20060530_FS_Women%27s%20HIV%20Prevention %20Control_en pdf (last accessed September 2007).

UNAIDS (2006c) 'Support women caregivers, fight AIDS', Geneva and Washington DC: UNAIDS, available at: http://data.unaids.org/pub/ FactSheet/2006/20060719_GCWA_FS_Support_Women_Caregivers_en.pdf (last accessed September 2007).

USAID (2003) 'Adding Family Planning to PMTCT Sites Increases the Benefits of PMTCT', Issue Brief: Population and Reproductive Health, October 2003, Wasington DC: USAID, available at: www.usaid.gov/ our_work/global_health/pop/techareas/familyplanning/fppmtct.pdf (last accessed September 2007).

Weissman, A., J. Cocker, L. Sherburne, M. B. Powers, R. Lovich, and M. Mukaka (2006) 'Cross-generational relationships: using a "Continuum of Volition" in HIV prevention work among young people', *Gender & Development* 14 (1): 81–94.

Welbourn, A. (2006) 'Sex, life and the female condom: some views of HIV positive women', *Reproductive Health Matters* 14 (28): 32–40.

WHO (2005) 'Mental Health and HIV-AIDS' series, Geneva: WHO, available at: www.who.int/mental_health/resources/mh_hiv_aids/en/ (last accessed September 2007).

Notes

1 For further reading in these areas, see the resources section.

2 One notable exception is the Movement of Men Against AIDS in Kenya: www.mmaak.org/ (last accessed September 2007).

3 See ICW Newsletter 37 (www.icw.org/files/ICW%20English%2037%20 web.pdf) and 'Male circumcision doesn't affect women's HIV risk' (www.aidsmap.com/en/news/863ED8A3-78C8-4C9C-BF22-FA0685E5D140.asp) for information about the issues surrounding HIV and male circumcision (both sites last accessed September 2007).

4 There are parallels here with attitudes towards sex before marriage for girls or boys, or towards divorce for men or women: in all cases males who break socially ascribed moral codes are let off more lightly than females.

5 You can access the call to action at www.worldywca.info/index.php/ ywca/world_council_iws/iws_women_s_summit/call_to_action/call_to _action (last accessed September 2007). The leadership of certain women has also been significant in changing attitudes within the women's move-ment. These include Musimbi Kanyoro, former Secretary General of the World YWCA, Mary Robinson, former Irish President and former head of the UN High Commission for Human Rights, who is patron of ICW, and Noerine Kaleeba, whose husband died of AIDS-related illnesses, and who started TASO, the first AIDS care organisation in Africa. There are also key HIV-positive women who have made huge changes in the world around them: see various ICW newsletters and the last section of this conclusion.

6 See for instance the autumn 2006 issue of Exchange on HIV/AIDS, sexuality, and gender, guest edited by ICW, for a discussion of the ABC prevention model, available at: www.icw.org/node/252 (last accessed September 2007).

7 See, for instance, two reports published by Christian Aid: 'Abstinence hurts' (www.christianaid.org.uk/stoppoverty/hiv/stories/abstinence.aspx) and 'Dying to learn: young people, HIV and the churches', available at: www.christianaid.org.uk/Images/dyingtolearn_tcm15-21616.pdf (both last accessed September 2007).

8 The Catholic international development NGO CAFOD, however, has spoken out in favour of promoting condom use as a means of preventing HIV, in the face of considerable criticism from the Vatican. See www.caritas.org/jumpNews.asp?idLang=ENG&idUser=0&id Channel=109&idNews=2173 (last accessed September 2007).

9 It is perfectly possible for a woman who is HIV-positive to give birth to a baby who is HIV-negative, provided she receives appropriate care and support. See www.hivandhepatitis.com/2007icr/ias/docs/073107_e.html for latest guidelines for discordant couples (i.e. where one partner is HIV-positive and the other is HIV-negative) who wish to have a baby without risk of infection either for the baby or the HIV-negative partner.

10 Thanks to Buck Buckingham of PEPFAR Kenya for this apt phrase.

11 More on this can be read on the ICW website (www.icw.org) as well as in the interview with gender and HIV expert and current UNFPA Deputy Executive Director Purnima Mane, available at: www.unaids.org/en/ MediaCentre/PressMaterials/FeatureStory/20070308_Interview_Purnima_ IWD2007.asp (last accessed September 2007).

12 There is also evidence, published by USAID in 2003, that providing comprehensive family-planning services, to enable women to avoid unplanned pregnancies, would be more cost-effective than provision of prevention of mother-to-child transmission (PMTCT) services to HIV-positive pregnant women. See USAID 2003.

13 See also ICW testing policy paper (www.icw.org/node/227), and Newsletter 37 (www.icw.org/files/ICW%20English%2037%20web.pdf) (both sites last accessed September 2007).

14 See www.icw.org/publications under 'Treatment Mappings' for three country studies (2006).

15 For more information about the Quality of Care model in relation to health-care provision in general, see WHO Gender, Women and Health Department: 'Gender Analysis in Health': a review of selected tools, WHO 2002, available at: www.who.int/gender/documents/en/ Gender.analysis.pdf (last accessed September 2007).

16 Increasing numbers of HIV-positive women are developing cervical cancer, and they seem to be particularly prone to abnormal cytology (Chirenje *et al.* 2001; ICW 2007b).

17 Personal communication, April 2005.

18 'A randomized controlled trial (RCT) is a scientific procedure most commonly used in testing medicines or medical procedures…Clinical RCTs involve allocating treatments to subjects at random.', http://en.wikipedia.org/wiki/Randomized_controlled_trial (last accessed September 2007).

19 For more discussion on the use of different research methods in the context of gender and development, see *Gender & Development* 15 (2) July 2007.

20 See www.sehn.org/precaution.html for an explanation of the Precautionary Principle in relation to scientific and environmental policies and practices in general (last accessed September 2007).

21 Family Health International (2007) 'How does HIV therapy affect hormonal contraception?, *Network* 24(1), www.fhi.org/en/RH/Pubs/ Network/v24_1/nt2415.htm (last accessed February 2008).

22 For more information on the need to reduce the cost of ARVs and to promote the production of generic drugs, please read the many documents available on the ICW and GNP+ websites – www.icw.org and www.gnpplus.net (both last accessed February 2008).

23 See www.timetodeliver.org/?p=266 (last accessed September 2007).

24 For examples of the challenges faced by HIV-positive people working in large institutions, see the website for 'UN+', the group for UN staff members who are openly HIV-positive: www.unplus.org.

25 WHO's announcement that it has agreed in principle to integrating gender analysis and actions into its work is most welcome but long overdue. How long it will take for this policy to be translated into practice within its organisational structure and in its work remains to be seen (see www.who.int/gender/mainstreaming/integrating_gender/en/index.html, last accessed September 2007).

26 The Treatment Action Campaign, mentioned by Sisonke Msimang in her chapter, is one group that fits this description. See www.tac.org.za/slideshow/SSMonalisa/small.html (last accessed September 2007).

Resources

Compiled by Joanna Hoare

This section presents useful resources for further study under the following headings:

- Education
- Gender violence
- HIV and young women
- Human rights
- Lesbian, gay, bisexual, and transgender (LGBT)
- Livelihoods
- Overcoming stigma
- Prevention
- Sex work
- Tools to integrate gender analysis into HIV and AIDS programmes
- Training resources
- Working with men
- General resources
- Organisations

Education

Deadly Inertia: A Cross Country Study of Educational Responses to HIV/AIDS (2005), Global Campaign for Education, PO Box 521733, Saxonwold, Johannesburg, 2132, South Africa, tel: +27 (0)11 447 4111, fax: +27 (0)11 447 4138, email: info@campaignforeducation.org, website: www.campaignforeducation.org
Available online at: www.campaignforeducation.org/resources/Nov2005/ENGLISHdeadlyinertia.pdf

Bringing together research in over 18 countries, this report finds that ministries of education are failing to provide an effective educational response to HIV and AIDS; one that could help children to protect themselves from HIV infection, as well as supporting children and teachers affected by HIV and AIDS. The international donor community has also failed to deliver leadership and political commitment. While the report does not have a specific gender focus, it does deal with how current teaching on HIV and lifeskills is failing girls and boys, and provides specific recommendations as to how this could be improved.

Letting Them Fail: Government Neglect and the Right to Education for Children Affected by AIDS (2005), Human Rights Watch, 350 Fifth Avenue, 34th floor, New York, NY 10118-3299 USA, tel: 1-(212) 290-4700, fax: 1-(212) 736-1300, email: hrwnyc@hrw.org
Available online at: http://hrw.org/reports/2005/africa1005/africa1005.pdf

Based on interviews with children and their caregivers in Kenya, Uganda, and South Africa, this report argues that governments are failing to address the enormous barriers to accessing education faced by children affected by HIV. These include inability to pay direct and indirect school fees; neglect, abuse, and exploitation at the hands of unscrupulous family members and foster carers; and having to drop out of school to care for sick relatives. The report highlights the particular vulnerability of girls affected by HIV to sexual abuse and exploitation.

Gender violence

Intimate Partner Violence and HIV/AIDS (2004), Department of Gender, Women and Health at the World Health Organization (WHO), Information Bulletin Series No.1, FCH/GWH, Batiment X, WHO, Avenue Appia 20, 1211 Geneva 27, Switzerland, fax: + 41 22 791 1585, email: genderandhealth@who.int, website: www.who.int/gender
Available online at: www.who.int/gender/violence/en/vawinformation brief.pdf

This information leaflet by WHO presents evidence on how violence against women and girls in its different forms increases their risk of HIV infection and undermines AIDS control efforts. It focuses on the links between violence against women and girls by intimate partners, and HIV.

Sexual violence in conflict settings and the risk of HIV (2004), Department of Gender, Women and Health, WHO. (Please see previous entry for contact details).
Available online at: www.who.int/gender/en/infobulletinconflict.pdf

This is the second in the series of information bulletins by WHO on the links between violence against women and their vulnerability to HIV. It focuses on the sexual violence that women and girls face in conflict settings and their increased risks of acquiring HIV as a result.

Show us the money: is violence against women on the HIV&AIDS funding agenda? (2007), written by Susanna T. Fried, ActionAid for the Women Won't Wait Campaign, ActionAid USA, 1420 K Street, NW, Suite 900, Washington DC 20005, USA, tel: +1-202-835-1240, fax: +1-202-835-1244. Available online at: www.womenwontwait.org/images/stories/Show %20Us%20The%20Money%20Full%20Report.pdf

This report analyses the policies, programming, and funding patterns of the largest public donors in relation to HIV, AIDS, and violence against women: the Global Fund to Fight AIDS, Tuberculosis and Malaria; the President's Emergency Fund for AIDS Relief (PEPFAR/US); the UK Department for International Development (DFID); and the World Bank and UNAIDS (the Joint UN Programme on HIV/AIDS). The report concludes that the major donors are still failing to consider violence against women as an integral aspect of the response to HIV, and as a consequence, are not providing consistent funding for such work. Among the list of recommendations are that donors should develop clear policy frameworks that give priority to violence against women and girls, HIV, and AIDS, and the inter-linkages between them.

Women, HIV and Sexual Violence (2005), amFAR, the Foundation for AIDS Research, 120 Wall Street, 13th Floor, New York, NY 10005-3908, tel: +1 (212) 806-1600, fax: +1 (212) 806-1601 / c/o TREAT Asia, Exchange Tower, 21st Floor, Suite 2104, 388 Sukhumvit Road, Klongtoey, Bangkok 10110, Thailand, tel: +66 (0)2 663 7561, fax: +66 (0)2 663 7562 Available online at: www.amfar.org/binary-data/AMFAR_PUBLICATION/ download_file/44.pdf

Contributors to this monograph argue that sexual violence is a major factor in the growing HIV epidemic among women and girls, but one which has received little attention to date, particularly in the medical community. Contributions outline medical research, research with women who have survived sexual violence, the work of activists who are themselves HIV-positive and survivors of sexual violence, and programmes challenging acceptance of sexual violence in the UK, USA, Bolivia, and Rwanda. While designed to raise awareness of the links between gender violence and HIV in the medical community, the articles in this collection are written in accessible, non-scientific language, making them relevant to a much wider audience.

HIV and young women

Act Now! A Resource Guide for Young Women on HIV/AIDS (2002),
The Association for Women's Rights in Development (AWID) and the
United Nations Development Fund for Women (UNIFEM) (contact details
for UNIFEM given below under 'Organisations').
Available online at: www.awid.org/publications/ActNow.pdf

This booklet is the result of a three-week email discussion on 'Young
Women and HIV/AIDS', hosted by AWID and UNIFEM. The discussion
focused on the linkages between youth, gender, HIV, and AIDS. It also
explored the ways in which young people can participate in addressing
gender and youth issues in HIV and AIDS programmes. This booklet is
targeted at young women who are leaders in their communities. It provides
an overview of the online discussions, and highlights and profiles young
women's leadership on HIV. It also provides useful activities for those who
want to start campaigns to raise awareness and decrease the stigma
associated with HIV and AIDS in their communities.

If I kept it to myself: young women intervene in a world with AIDS (2006),
World YWCA, 16 Ancienne Route, 1218 Grand Saconnex, Geneva
Switzerland, tel: +41 22 929 6040, fax: +41 22 929 6044,
email: worldoffice@worldywca.org
Available online at: www.worldywca.info/index.php/ywca/
world_ywca/communications/resources/if_i_kept_it_to_myself

All over the world, young women are active as peer counsellors and
educators, caregivers, and as people living openly with HIV or AIDS. This
book seeks to document the experiences of some of these women, in order to
inspire others. With testimonies from young activists, it includes sections on
advocacy, education, care and support, media and communications, and
'pioneers'. These are supplemented with 'Tool boxes', containing ideas and
tips for practical action.

Women and Girls living with HIV/AIDS: Overview and Annotated Bibliography
(2007), by Emily Esplen, BRIDGE, Institute of Development Studies,
University of Sussex, Brighton BN1 9RE, UK, tel: +44 (0) 1273 606261,
fax: +44 (0) 1273 621202/691647, email: bridge@ids.ac.uk,
website: www.ids.ac.uk/bridge
Available online at: www.bridge.ids.ac.uk/reports/BB18_HIV.pdf

This report considers the specific challenges faced by women and girls
who are living with HIV and AIDS. Consisting of an overview, annotated
bibliography, and a contacts section, this covers a wide variety of topics,
including: access to care, treatment, and support; sexual and reproductive
rights; legal and economic rights; violence against HIV positive women;
and leadership, participation, and voice.

Human rights

Epidemic of Inequality: Women's Rights and HIV/AIDS in Botswana &
Swaziland, An Evidence-Based Report on the Effects of Gender Inequity, Stigma
and Discrimination (2007), Physicians for Human Rights, 2 Arrow Street,
Suite 301, Cambridge, MA 02138, USA, tel: +1 617 301 4200,
fax: +1 617 301 4250, website: http://physiciansforhumanrights.org
Available online at: http://physiciansforhumanrights.org/library/
documents/reports/botswana-swaziland-report.pdf

Botswana and Swaziland have the highest rates of HIV prevalence in the
world. The legal, social, economic, and cultural discrimination that women
face in both countries contributes to their disproportionate vulnerability to
HIV infection. On the basis of evidence collected through community
surveys and interviews with people living with HIV or AIDS, this detailed
report argues that HIV interventions that are focused solely on individual
behaviour will not address the factors creating vulnerability to HIV for
women and men in Botswana and Swaziland, nor protect the rights and
assure the well-being of those living with HIV or AIDS. Rather, the
governments of the two countries must act to protect the rights of women.

Male circumcision and HIV prevention: a human rights and public health
challenge (2007), Canadian HIV/AIDS Legal Network, 1240 Bay Street,
Suite 600, Toronto, Ontario M5R 2A7, Canada, tel: +1 416 595 1666,
fax: +1 416 595 0094, email: info@aidslaw.ca, website: www.aidslaw.ca.
Available online at: www.aidslaw.ca/publications/interfaces/
downloadFile.php?ref=1128

Recent research has concluded that male circumcision can lead to
significant reduction of HIV risk for men. This article identifies and
discusses the important human-rights questions that should be taken into
account in the development of policy guidelines for national governments
seeking to 'scale up' male circumcision as a prevention method. The author
suggests that education and counselling provided as part of such a scale-up
of services would provide an excellent opportunity to address issues
concerning the subordination of women, provided they are appropriately
designed and funded.

Not Separate, Still Unequal: The Beijing Agreement and the Feminization of
HIV/AIDS (2005), Adrienne Germain and Jennifer Kidwell, *American*
Sexuality Magazine 3 (2).
Available online at: www.iwhc.org/resources/asmapril2005.cfm

This article explains how the full implementation of the Beijing Platform
for Action by governments would help to reduce women's and girls' greater
vulnerability to HIV. It urges greater investment in sexual and reproductive
health education and greater provision of health services by governments.

Women, HIV/AIDS and human rights (2004), Amnesty International, International Secretariat, Peter Benenson House, 1 Easton Street, London, WC1X 0DW, UK, website: www.amnesty.org
Available online at: http://web.amnesty.org/library/Index/ENGACT770842004

This paper provides a human-rights analysis of the gender-specific factors which put women at risk of contracting HIV. It also analyses the consequences for women of contracting HIV. The evidence highlights that violence against women and other forms of gender-based discrimination increase women's likelihood of contracting HIV, and that gender-based discrimination also hinders women's access to prevention methods and to treatment. It argues that a rights-based approach is needed to effectively tackle the pandemic, its causes and consequences, and that international co-operation is needed to tackle the global inequalities surrounding the prevalence of HIV and the lack of access to treatment.

Women's Human Rights related to Health-Care Services in the Context of HIV/AIDS (2004), Gillian MacNaughton, World Health Organization, Health and Human Rights Working Paper Series No 5.
Available online at: www.who.int/hhr/information/en/Series_5_womenshealthcarerts_MacNaughtonFINAL.pdf

The paper addresses the difficulties that people, especially women and girls in Southern countries, face in seeking HIV and AIDS-related health care. It begins by examining the impact of HIV on women and girls, including their vulnerability to infection and the discrimination they face after infection. It also looks at the increased burden women and girls carry in caring for family members who fall ill. The paper then explains the international response to HIV, presenting the history of the United Nations' political commitments on HIV-related issues. Also included is an outline of international legal obligations arising from international human-rights treaties. The final section of the paper discusses legal issues central to HIV health-care services: voluntary HIV testing, medical confidentiality, HIV-related discrimination in health-care services, and the right to treatment.

Lesbian, gay, bisexual, and transgender (LGBT)

Durban Lesbian and Gay Community and Health Centre: Gender HIV/AIDS Analysis (2005), Margaret Roper and Eric Richardson, the Joint Oxfam HIV and AIDS Programme in South Africa (Managing Affiliate – Oxfam Australia, 132 Leicester Street, Carlton VIC 3053, Australia, tel: +61 (0)3 9289 9444, fax: +61 (0)3 9347 1983).
Available online at: www.oxfam.org.au/world/africa/south_africa/DurbanGenderAnalysis.pdf

This report by the Joint Oxfam HIV and AIDS Programme (JOHAP) 2005 looks at how the Durban Lesbian and Gay Community and Health Centre in KwaZulu-Natal, South Africa is working with lesbian, gay, bisexual, and transgender communities on HIV prevention, treatment, and care.

International Lesbian and Gay Association (ILGA): resources on HIV and AIDS
Available online at: www.ilga.org/files_target.asp?FileCategoryID=55

This 'virtual library' contains a small selection of materials on HIV, AIDS, and LGBT issues, published by ILGA and other organisations.

Off the map: how HIV/AIDS programming is failing same-sex practising people in Africa (2007), International Gay and Lesbian Human Rights Commission, 80 Maiden Lane, Suite 1505, New York, NY 10038, USA, tel: +1 212 268 8040, fax: +1 212 430 6060, email: iglhrc@iglhrc.org, website: www.iglhrc.org
Available online at: www.iglhrc.org/files/iglhrc/otm/Off%20The%20Map.pdf

Off the map explores the ways in which governments, donors, and NGOs are denying basic human-rights protection to same-sex practising Africans, potentially jeopardising overall responses to HIV in the process. The report shows that same-sex practising men and women are at increased risk of contracting HIV not solely because of bio-sexual vulnerabilities, but because the widespread criminalisation and denial of same-sex desire and practice prevents their access to effective HIV prevention, voluntary counselling and testing, treatment, and care. Chapters on 'Denial and homophobia', 'What we know about same-sex practising people and HIV in Africa', and 'The impact of African government policies on the sexual health of same-sex practising people' (among others) are followed by a list of recommendations.

Livelihoods

HIV/AIDS and the Environment: impacts of AIDS and ways to reduce them (2007), Judy Oglethorpe and Nancy Gelman, World Wildlife Fund, 1250 Twenty-Fourth Street, N.W. P.O. Box 97180, Washington, DC 20090-7180, USA, tel: +1 (202) 293-4800, website: www.worldwildlife.org
Available online at: http://worldwildlife.org/phe/pubs/hivaids.pdf

In addition to its tragic impacts on families and communities, AIDS is also affecting the environment through its impact on rural livelihoods, natural-resource management, and land use. Topics covered include loss of traditional knowledge about the sustainable management of natural resources, land grabbing, and how current methods of natural-resource extraction (such as logging and fishing) are helping to spread HIV, through their reliance on migrant labour. Aimed at those working in conservation, this pamphlet outlines ways that conservation programmes can mainstream HIV into their work, and how organisations can support staff, and help them to avoid infection.

HIV/AIDS and Food Security webportal
Available online at: www.fao.org/hivaids/

Resources provided via this web portal focus on the distinct impact HIV and AIDS has on food security and rural livelihoods. Themes on the site include the impact of HIV and AIDS on food security in relation to issues of poverty, nutrition, gender, knowledge, and labour. A variety of publications are available (free to download) on topics such as agriculture, fisheries, gender and equity, knowledge and capacity, methodological approaches, and policy and strategy.

HIV/AIDS, Gender Inequality and the Agricultural Sector (2004), Interagency Coalition on AIDS and Development (ICAD), 1 Nicholas Street, Suite 726, Ottawa, ON K1N 7B7, Canada.
Available online at: www.icad-cisd.com/pdf/publications/Gender_Inequality_Agriculture_FINAL.pdf

This report discusses how agriculture can play an important role in responses to HIV and AIDS by reducing poverty and improving food security. It argues that for rural households that are affected by the epidemic, agricultural and food-security programmes are key to helping them achieve self-sufficiency. These guidelines give a summary of existing information related to the links between HIV, AIDS, gender inequality, and agricultural development. They provide recommendations on how these factors can be taken into account when developing, reviewing, and implementing agricultural programmes in Southern Africa.

HIV/AIDS, gender and rural livelihoods in sub-Saharan Africa: An overview and annotated bibliography (2005), Tanja R. Mueller, Wageningen Academic Publishers, P.O Box 220, 6700 AE Wageningen, The Netherlands, website: www.WageningenAcademic.com, email: sales@WageningenAcademic.com

This book explores the links between gender, HIV, and AIDS in sub-Saharan Africa. In particular, it focuses on women in rural areas and the gender-specific impacts of the epidemic on them as mothers and caregivers as well as food producers. The author argues that existing cultural norms and unequal power relations in sub-Saharan Africa make women more vulnerable to HIV infection. At the same time, their limited access to and ownership of land makes it difficult for them to ensure their families have enough food to eat. The author emphasises that a transformation in unequal gender relations is crucial to address these problems.

Overcoming stigma

HIV-Related Stigma, Discrimination and Human Rights Violations: Case studies of successful programmes (2005), UNAIDS Best Practice Collection, UNAIDS (contact details given below under 'Organisations').
Available online at: http://data.unaids.org/publications/irc-pub06/JC999-HumRightsViol_en.pdf

Stigma and discrimination play key roles in fuelling the transmission of HIV, and in increasing the negative impacts associated with the epidemic. In this way, stigma is closely associated with the denial and violation of human rights that many HIV-positive people experience. Women are more likely than men to suffer from stigmatisation and discrimination as a result of their HIV status, a situation closely linked to their unequal status in society and sexual 'double standards' that punish women for sexual activity. This paper presents case studies of programmes in countries in Southern Africa, East Asia, Latin America, Eastern Europe, South Asia, and East Africa, which have challenged HIV-related stigma in innovative and successful ways, either as part of targeted interventions, or of more holistic projects.

Understanding and Challenging HIV Stigma: Toolkit for Action (revised edition) (2007), International HIV/AIDS Alliance/Academy for Educational Development/International Center for Research on Women (contact details for International HIV/AIDS Alliance given below under 'Organisations').
Available online at: www.aidsalliance.org/custom_asp/publications/view.asp?publication_ id=255&language=en

This toolkit was originally developed from a research project on HIV-related stigma and discrimination in Ethiopia, Tanzania, and Zambia, with the involvement of staff from over 50 NGOs in these countries. It consists of participatory educational exercises for use in raising awareness and promoting action to challenge HIV-related stigma. It is designed to be adapted for use with different target groups, including community groups and AIDS professionals. Facilitators are encouraged to pick and choose from a range of different methods and modules, which cover issues such as 'Naming the problem', 'Sex, morality, blame and shame', and 'Caring for PLWA in the family'. In addition to those included in the original toolkit, new modules address stigma as it relates to treatment, children and young people, and men who have sex with men.

Prevention

The effectiveness of condoms in preventing HIV transmission (2005), amFAR, the Foundation for AIDS Research, 120 Wall Street, 13th Floor, New York, NY 10005-3908, tel: +1 (212) 806-1600, fax: +1 (212) 806-1601/
c/o TREAT Asia, Exchange Tower, 21st Floor, Suite 2104, 388 Sukhumvit Road, Klongtoey, Bangkok 10110, Thailand, tel: +66 (0)2 663 7561,
fax: +66 (0)2 663 7562
Available online at: www.amfar.org/binary-data/AMFAR_PPOLICY_
BINARY/binary_file/11.pdf

This short policy brief provides a summary of the scientific evidence supporting the use of male and female condoms as an effective way of preventing HIV transmission, particularly when they are used as part of a comprehensive prevention programme. In this way, it refutes many of the claims made in current US policy documents, which emphasise a lack of condom effectiveness in HIV prevention.

New approaches to HIV prevention: accelerating research and ensuring future access (2006), Global HIV Prevention Working Group,
email: info@globalhivprevention.org, website: globalhivprevention.org.
Available online at: www.globalhivprevention.org/pdfs/New%20P
revention%20Approaches.pdf

This report summarises the current state of HIV prevention research. It makes recommendations to increase research on promising new HIV prevention methods, and to ensure rapid access to new tools and strategies as soon as they are proven effective. Subjects covered include different methods currently under consideration, such as male circumcision and microbicides, ethical considerations in clinical trials, and engaging communities in prevention research. The report also highlights the potential importance of developing prevention methods that could be initiated and used by women, with or without their partner's knowledge.

Sex work

HIV and sexually transmitted infection prevention among sex workers in Eastern Europe and Central Asia (2006), UNAIDS Best Practice Collection, UNAIDS (contact details given below under 'Organisations').
Available online at: http://data.unaids.org/Publications/IRC-pub07/JC1212-HIVPrevEasternEurCentrAsia_en.pdf

The number of people infected with HIV in Eastern Europe and Central Asia has increased dramatically in recent years, and commercial sex work has become an important factor in many countries' epidemics. This report describes the experiences of, and challenges faced by, different organisations dealing with HIV and sexually transmitted infection prevention for sex workers in Kyrgyzstan, Russia, Ukraine, Poland, and Hungary. It mentions the importance of tailoring HIV prevention and support programmes to specific needs of sex workers, and of adopting a broad-based approach that encourages vulnerable groups to gain control of their health.

Practical guidelines for delivering health services to sex workers (2003), The European Network for HIV/STD prevention in Prostitution (EUROPAP).
Available online at: www.europap.net/dl/guidelines/layoutENG.pdf

These guidelines are designed for use by health and social workers. They are for the most part practical, and deal with a wide range of issues, and include an extensive section on HIV and sexually transmitted infections. Throughout, the importance of involving sex workers in the design and implementation of programmes is emphasised.

Tools to integrate gender analysis into HIV and AIDS programmes

Gender and HIV/AIDS: Guidelines for integrating a gender focus into NGO work on HIV/AIDS (2002), ActionAid, Agency for Co-operation and Research in Development (ACORD), and Save the Children, Save the Children Publications, c/o NBN International, Estover Road, Plymouth, PL6 7PY, UK, tel: +44 (0)1752 202301, fax: +44 (0)1752 202333,
email: orders@nbninternational.com
Available online at www.acordinternational.org/index.php/downloads/Gender_and_HIV/AIDS%3A_Guidelines_for_integrating_a_gender_focus_into_NGO_work_on_HIV/AIDS

This is a revised and updated version of the guidelines produced by three UK development agencies to assist staff of international and local NGOs to carry out research on HIV, AIDS, and gender. It is also intended to help them plan HIV and AIDS programmes more effectively. It provides information on the relationship between gender and the spread of HIV. It also provides frameworks to help identify and analyse the links between gender, HIV, and other social, economic, and political factors. The guidelines feature case studies that highlight different types of participatory methods that can be used while working on gender and HIV. The final section includes recent resources and websites with further information on the issues and approaches that are discussed in the guidelines.

How Gender-Sensitive Are Your HIV and Family Planning Services? A tool for self-assessment (2002), International Planned Parenthood Federation, Western Hemisphere Region, 120 Wall Street, 9th Floor, New York, NY 10005-3902, tel: 001 (0) 212-248-6400, fax: 001 (0) 212-248-4221, email: info@ippfwhr.org, website: www.ippfwhr.org
Available online at: www.ippfwhr.org/publications/download/monographs/gender_continuum.pdf

This HIV/Gender Continuum is a tool to enable organisations to assess how responsive their services and programmes are to gender issues related to HIV prevention. The tool is written from a rights-based perspective on sexual and reproductive health. Programmes that fall to the left of the Continuum need major changes, programmes that fall in the middle are moving in a gender-sensitive direction, and programmes that fall to the right are model programmes.

NGO Strategies for Gender Mainstreaming in HIV/AIDS Programming (2004), Rebecca Tiessen, paper presented at the International Studies Association Conference, Montreal, March 2004.
Available online at: http://media-cyber.law.harvard.edu/blogs/gems/politicshiv/tiessen.pdf

This paper argues that the technical solutions employed by NGOs to mainstream gender fail to address the attitudes, norms, and behaviours which reinforce gender inequality. The author stresses that what is needed to tackle HIV is transformative planning by NGOs, as well as change in attitudes and behaviour. The paper discusses successful examples of such strategies, which have the potential to make real change in the way in which development NGOs think about gender mainstreaming. The emphasis is on how these innovative approaches can facilitate women's empowerment.

Resource pack on gender and HIV/AIDS (2005), UNAIDS/KIT Publishers, Royal Tropical Institute, Mauritskade 63, 1092 AD Amsterdam, The Netherlands, tel: +31 20 56 88 711, fax: +31 20 66 84 579.
Available online at: www.kit.nl/smartsite.shtml?&id=SINGLEPUBLICATION&ItemID=1868&AdvancedSearch=False

This resource pack analyses the impact of unequal gender relations on the different aspects of the HIV epidemic, and makes recommendations for effective programme and policy options. An expert review paper provides a gender and rights-based conceptual framework for integrating gender into HIV and AIDS programmes. This is accompanied by 16 fact sheets, each providing concise information on a different topic, such as male and female condoms, young people, and the prevention of mother-to-child transmission, along with a list of useful references.

Training resources

'Auntie Stella': teenagers talk about sex, life and relationships, Adolescent Reproductive Health Project (ARHEP), Training and Research Support Centre (TARSC), 47 Van Praagh Avenue, Milton Park, Harare, Zimbabwe, tel: 263 4 705108, fax: 263 4 737220, email: tarsc@mweb.co.zw
Available online at: www.tarsc.org/auntstella/index.html

'Auntie Stella' is an activity pack originally developed in Zimbabwe, and designed to help teenagers discuss and obtain information on a wide range of issues, including HIV and other sexually transmitted infections, and gender relations. The pack consists of a set of over 30 'question letters', of the type that might be written to an agony aunt or uncle in a newspaper or magazine. Young people are encouraged to discuss the contents of each letter, prompted by a set of questions that accompany it, and then turn to 'Auntie Stella's' reply for expert information and suggestions about how to apply any new knowledge in real life, followed by discussion on ways to change their behaviour. The pack is available online and in a print version.

HIV, AIDS, & Islam: A Workshop Manual Based on Compassion, Responsibility and Justice (2007), Positive Muslims, P.O. Box 13127, Mowbray, 7705, Cape Town, South Africa, tel: + 27 21 448 7643, fax: + 27 21 448 8241, email: info@positivemuslims.org.za
Available online at: www.coreinitiative.org/Resources/Publications/CORE_PM.pdf

This training manual is designed for those working to raise awareness of HIV within Muslim communities, and consists of a series of workshop activities. These provide participants with basic information about HIV and its prevalence in Muslim communities, and prompt them to discuss issues of stigmatisation, social responsibility, and morality. The manual specifically addresses the links between gender, poverty, and the spread and treatment of HIV and AIDS, with sections on 'Women, HIV and AIDS', 'The Shari'ah, Muslim Society, and Gender', and 'AIDS, Sex, and Sexuality'.

Ideas for working with girls: materials on violence against women, rights, health & sexuality, advocacy and more..., International Women's Tribune Centre (ITWC), 777 United Nations Plaza, New York, NY 10017, USA, tel: +1 212 687-8633, fax: +1 212 661-2704, email: iwtc@iwtc.org, website: www.iwtc.org/6774.html

This CD contains material such as free games, training manuals, and workshop guides for teachers, trainers, and development workers who are working for and with girls. It includes interactive and participatory training guides and resources on rights, empowerment, violence against women and girls, HIV, sexuality and reproductive health, and leadership development. The CD is free and can be ordered from the address given above. Its contents can also be downloaded from the website.

Program H, Instituto Promundo, Rua México, 31/1502, Centro, Rio de Janeiro – RJ, 20031-144, Brazil, tel/fax: +55 (21) 2544-3114, email: promundo@promundo.org.br, website: www.promundo.org.br/ (English), www.promundo.org.br/15699?locale=pt_BR (Portuguese)

Program H encourages young men to question traditional norms associated with masculinity and promotes both discussion and reflection about the costs of traditional masculinity, as well as the advantages of gender-equitable behaviours. Originally developed for use in Brazil, but widely replicated elsewhere, it focuses particularly on challenging violence against women, and encouraging young men to take responsibility for their own sexual and reproductive health. A recent programme evaluation (www.promundo.org.br/Downloads/PDF/Relatorio%20Final%20Horizons%20(ingles).pdf) found that young men who had taken part had more positive attitudes and behaviour regarding protecting themselves from HIV and other sexually transmitted infections, and were more likely to use condoms. In addition to information about the programme, and Instituto Promundo's other activities, the website allows visitors to download or purchase the Program H training materials, available in Portuguese, Spanish, and English.

Stepping Stones: A training package in HIV/AIDS, communication and relationship skills (1995), Alice Welbourn, ActionAid, London, available to order from TALC, PO Box 49, St Albans, Herts, AL1 5TX, UK, tel: +44 (0) 1727 853869, fax: +44 (0) 1727 846852, email: info@talcuk.org / e-talc@talcuk.org, website: www.talcuk.org/catalog/
More information on *Stepping Stones* is available at www.steppingstonesfeedback.org/

This is a training pack on gender, HIV, communication, and relationship skills, for use with whole communities. The aim of the training is to support older and younger males and females, separately and together, to explore their own issues in a community-wide, holistic response which recognises the key role of consistent mutual support in the process of sustained change of any kind. The package consists of a manual for trainers (and an optional workshop video). Planned originally for use in communities throughout sub-Saharan Africa, the package has now also been adapted for use elsewhere in Africa, in Asia, the Pacific, Eastern Europe, Latin America, and the Caribbean. A recent evaluation by the South Africa Medical Research Council (2007) reported a reduction in gender-based violence and sexual risk-taking among young men who had been through the *Stepping Stones* programme, as well as a reduction in the transmission of sexually transmitted infections. The evaluation is available online at www.mrc.ac.za/policybriefs/steppingstones.pdf.

Working with men

Gender Analysis of Targeted AIDS Intervention (TAI) (2005), Graham Lindegger and Justin Maxwell, the Joint Oxfam HIV/AIDS Programme in South Africa (Managing Affiliate – Oxfam Australia. See entry above in 'LGBT' for contact details).
Available online at: www.oxfam.org.au/world/africa/south_africa/AIDS GenderAnalysis.pdf

This is the first in a series of reports on the Joint Oxfam HIV and AIDS Programme (JOHAP) 2005. It looks at the work of the Targeted AIDS Intervention (TAI) Project, an NGO in South Africa that offers HIV education and training to men and boys in particular. TAI's work is based on the understanding that HIV must be understood as a function of how 'masculinity' is thought of and demonstrated in behaviour. This report examines how TAI are working with young men and boys to try and change their notions of masculinity and therefore alter behaviour that increases their risk of HIV infection.

HIV and Men who have Sex with Men in Asia and the Pacific (2006), UNAIDS Best Practice Collection, UNAIDS (contact details given below under 'Organisations').
Available online at: http://data.unaids.org/Publications/IRC-pub07/ JC901-MSM-AsiaPacific_en.pdf

This comprehensive report records the experiences of six HIV prevention programmes working with men who have sex with men in Bangladesh, India, Indonesia, the Philippines, Hong Kong, and New Zealand. In addition to providing detailed accounts of the individual programmes, the report includes a 'lessons learned' section covering four themes: working with governments and health authorities; working with mainstream communities; health services; and outreach activities. While encouraging readers to adapt and use these lessons in their own work with men who have sex with men, the authors urge caution, highlighting that an assessment of individual situations and environments is crucial before adopting any of the ideas suggested, as some may be counter-productive or even dangerous in some environments.

Implementing HIV/AIDS/STI peer education for uniformed services (2003), UNAIDS (contact details given below under 'Organisations').
Available online at: http://data.unaids.org/Publications/IRC-pub05/ JC928-EngagingUniServices-PeerEd_en.pdf

Men (and women) serving in armed forces are at particular risk of contracting HIV, and of passing it on to members of the civilian populations with which they come into contact. This training pack contains participatory group exercises designed to de-sensitise sexual issues, help participants to assess risk, and to enhance communication within relationships, with the aim of changing attitudes and behaviour around sex, and encouraging uniformed services personnel to become advocates in the response to HIV. In addition to sections on topics such as risk assessment, condom use, and professional contact, there is a section on gender, coercion, and sexual violence. While designed for use with soldiers, this pack could be useful for others working in predominantly male environments.

'Man hunt intimacy: man clean bathroom': women, sexual pleasure, gender violence and HIV (2006), Alice Welbourn, *IDS Bulletin* 37 (5), Institute of Development Studies, Brighton, BN1 9RE, UK, tel: +44 (0)1273 606261, fax: +44 (0)1273 621202, email: ids@ids.ac.uk, website: www.ids.ac.uk
Available online at: www.steppingstonesfeedback.org/downloads/ Welbourn_ManHuntIntimacy_2006.pdf

This short article explores the links between sexuality, gender violence, and HIV in heterosexual relationships. Using examples from a range of workshop contexts, it argues that if women and men are encouraged to discuss sex and sexuality openly, and if men are encouraged to recognise the sexual, emotional, and practical needs of their female partners, both men and women will be less likely to engage in unsafe sex, and more likely to have relationships that are free from violence, and equitable.

UNAIDS Policy Brief: HIV and sex between men (2006), UNAIDS (contact details given below under 'Organisations').
Available online at: http://data.unaids.org/Publications/IRC-pub07/ JC1269-PolicyBrief-MSM_en.pdf

This short policy brief outlines the main issues around HIV and sex between men, as well as presenting UNAIDS' policy position on the subject. In particular, it argues that HIV as it affects men who have sex with men should not be regarded as a discrete issue, but rather should be linked to the wider HIV epidemic, given that in many cases, men who have unprotected sex with men may also be having unprotected sex with female partners. The report concludes by calling for national governments to decriminalise homosexuality and to act against the stigma and discrimination that prevent so many men from accessing appropriate support and care, and prevent them exercising their right to protect themselves from HIV.

General resources

AIDSPortal
Available online at: www.aidsportal.org

AIDSPortal provides tools to support global collaboration and knowledge sharing among new and existing networks of people responding to the AIDS epidemic throughout the world. It has a dedicated section for those working on gender and HIV, with links to recent publications, and details of upcoming events. Topics covered include women's rights and HIV, men and masculinities, female-controlled prevention methods, and HIV and gender-based violence.

Breaking barriers: Effective communication for universal access to HIV prevention, treatment, care and support by 2010 (2006), Robin Vincent, Panos Global AIDS Programme, Panos Southern Africa, PO Box 39163, Plot 32A Leopards Hill Road, Woodlands, Lusaka, Zambia, tel: + 260 1 263 258, fax: + 260 1 261 039, email: general@panos.org.zm
Available online at: www.panos.org.uk/PDF/reports/breakingbarriers.pdf

This report argues that effective HIV and AIDS communication is vital, if the goal agreed in 2005 by the African Union, the UN Summit, and the G8 governments to attain universal access to HIV prevention, treatment, care, and support by 2010 is to be achieved. Communication approaches need to look beyond narrow, short-term interventions that focus on changing individual behaviour. Instead, we need to engage with the social and economic drivers of the epidemic, including gender inequality, in a way that is informed by the experiences and priorities of those most affected.

Civil Society Perspectives on HIV/AIDS Policy in Nicaragua, Senegal, Ukraine, the United States, and Vietnam (2007), Public Health Watch/Open Society Institute, 400 West 59th Street, New York, New York 10019, USA, tel: + 1 212 548 0600, email: phwinfo@sorosny.org
Available online at: www.soros.org/initiatives/health/focus/phw/articles_publications/publications/perspectives_20070626/civilsociety_20070626.pdf

This report argues that national governments and international agencies are continuing to ignore or exclude marginalised groups in their responses to HIV and AIDS. In particular, in the contexts of the five countries covered in this report, injecting drug users, sex workers, men who have sex with men, prisoners, and ethnic minorities are frequently excluded from participating in the design, implementation, and evaluation of national HIV and AIDS responses, with implications for their capacity to protect themselves from HIV, and access treatment if they need to do so. Civil-society groups have the necessary knowledge, experience, and access to these marginalised groups, to be able to articulate their perspectives. As such, national governments and international agencies should do more to integrate civil society into their policy design and implementation strategies.

Eldis Gender and HIV and AIDS resource pages
Available online at: www.eldis.org/go/topics/resource-guides/hiv-and-aids/gender

These web pages provide links to a wide range of papers, toolkits, manuals, and other resources on gender, HIV, and AIDS. Included are sections on women and girls, men, and a series of 'Key Issues' papers, which so far have covered violence against women and HIV, the female condom, and microbicides. Visitors can also subscribe to regular email updates on particular subjects of interest.

The greater involvement of people living with HIV (GIPA) (2007), UNAIDS (contact details given below under 'Organisations').
Available online at: http://data.unaids.org/pub/Report/2007/ JC1299-PolicyBrief-GIPA_en.pdf

People living with HIV should have the right to input into decision-making that will impact upon their lives. In addition, they have direct experience of the factors that make individuals and communities vulnerable to HIV infection. Their involvement in programme development and implementation and policy-making will improve the relevance, acceptability, and effectiveness of programmes, and is critical to halting and reversing the epidemic. This short document outlines UNAIDS' policy position on the greater involvement of people with HIV (GIPA), recommending actions for governments, organisations of people living with HIV, wider civil society and the private sector, and international partners.

How to be a 'proper' woman in the time of AIDS (2007), Katja Jassey and Stella Nyanzi, *Current African Issues* 34, The Nordic Africa Institute, P O Box 1703, SE-751 47 Uppsala, Sweden, tel: +46 18 56 22 00, fax: +46 18 56 22 90, email: nai@nai.uu.se
Available online at: www.nai.uu.se/publications/download.html/978-91-7106-574-2.pdf?id=25192

Written by two women who have worked in gender, HIV, and development for many years, this paper reflects on the messages contained within anti-HIV campaigns, and what they say about 'acceptable' gender roles and behaviour, marriage, and sexuality, asking why there is such an absence of messages that include, or would make sense to, people living with HIV. Drawing on interviews with women and men who talk about their experiences of love, sexuality, and relationships in the context of living with HIV, the authors also raise pertinent questions regarding who is accorded the 'right' to produce information and knowledge about HIV in the current climate.

Impacts of HIV/AIDS 2005–2025 in Papua New Guinea, Indonesia and East Timor: Final Report of HIV Epidemiological Modelling and Impact Study (2006), AusAID, GPO Box 887, Canberra ACT 2601, Australia, tel: +61 2 6206 4727, fax: +61 2 6206 4695
Available online at: www.ausaid.gov.au/publications/pdf/impacts_hiv.pdf

Drawing on the results of a study designed to predict the possible development and impact of the AIDS epidemic in Papua New Guinea, Indonesia, and East Timor, this lengthy report proposes three scenarios for each country. In the first, predications are given for the impact of the epidemic if HIV interventions remain at current levels; in the second, if they are increased to medium response; and in the third, if they are increased to high response. Part 2 of the report includes a comprehensive assessment of the current and predicted future economic and social impacts of the disease, including on gender relations. The interplay between gender, HIV, and other issues such as education, migration, and conflict, is also considered.

Mapping Multilateral Development Banks' Reproductive Health and HIV/AIDS Spending (2007), Suzanna Denis and Elaine Zuckerman, Gender Action, 1875 Connecticut Avenue NW, Suite 1012, Washington DC 20009, USA, tel: +1 202-587-5242, email: info@genderaction.org,
website: www.genderaction.org
Available online at: www.genderaction.org/images/Gender%20Action%20MDBs%20RH-AIDS.pdf

This report analyses the extent to which the Multilateral Development Banks (MDB) are meeting their commitments to promote reproductive health, prevent HIV, and treat AIDS. It analyses the quantity and quality of

MDB funding for these sectors during 2003–2006 and highlights how MDB and International Monetary Fund (IMF) policies undermine achieving the reproductive health and HIV and AIDS targets of the Millennium Development Goals (MDGs). The authors also state that MDB projects are failing to address gender issues adequately, in particular by overlooking men's involvement in reproductive health and rights, and by focusing primarily on maternal health, rather than sexual and reproductive health and rights.

Triple Jeopardy: Women and AIDS (1990/2004), Panos Publications, 9 White Lion Street London Nl 9PD, UK, tel: +44 20 7278 1111, fax: + 44 20 7278 0345, website: www.panos.org.uk
Available online at: www.panos.org.uk/images/books/TRIPLE%20 JEOPARDY%20WOMEN%20&%20AIDS.pdf

With an updated introduction written in 2004, this publication from the Panos Global AIDS Programme draws attention to the triple threat that women face from the AIDS pandemic as individuals, mothers, and carers. It stresses that gender inequality fuels HIV infection, that stigma and blame prevent many women from leaving relationships that put them at risk of HIV infection, and that HIV and AIDS worsen women's and girls' poverty and inequality.

UNIFEM's Gender and HIV/AIDS Web Portal
Available online at: www.genderandaids.org

UNIFEM, in collaboration with UNAIDS, has developed this gender, HIV, and AIDS web portal to provide up-to-date information on the HIV epidemic from a gender-aware perspective. The website aims to promote understanding, knowledge sharing, and action on HIV and AIDS as gender and human-rights issues. It provides research, studies and surveys, training materials, advocacy tools, speeches and presentations, current news, best practices, personal stories, campaign actions, and opinion pieces by leading commentators. Resources from the web portal's Electronic Library are also available on a CD, which can be obtained free of charge from unifem@genderandaids.org. This covers a range of topics including gender mainstreaming, HIV, and AIDS; gender, sexuality, and power relations; gender, human rights, HIV, and AIDS; prevention, treatment, and care; and legislation and policy. The CD includes a variety of materials in French and Spanish.

Women, Children, and HIV: resources for prevention and treatment
Available online at: http://womenchildrenhiv.org/

This extensive virtual library contains resources on the prevention and treatment of HIV infection in women and children, targeted at health workers, programme managers, and policy makers in resource-poor settings. While aimed at those who have a medical background, the website holds resources that are suitable for a more general audience as well. These include journal articles, a generic training pack on preventing mother-to-child transmissions, HIV country profiles, and a list of Top Forty Resources for Starting HIV Prevention, Care, and Treatment Programs in Developing Countries.

Organisations

Global Campaign for Microbicides, c/o PATH, 1800 K Street NW, Washington D.C. 20006, USA, tel: +1 (202) 822-0033, fax: +1 (202) 457-1466, email: info@global-campaign.org, website: www.global-campaign.org/

The Global Campaign for Microbicides is a network of over 280 NGOs which campaigns to raise awareness and mobilise political support for increased funding for microbicide research, and for the female condom and other cervical barrier methods of preventing HIV and other sexually transmitted infections. Through its advocacy, research, and policy-analysis work, it aims to accelerate the development of, and increase access to microbicides, while protecting the needs and interests of users. The organisation has a particular focus on ensuring that women's rights are upheld in any clinical trials. The website provides information about microbicides and other methods of protection, research ethics in the context of trialling microbicides, and access to a range of useful publications.

The Global Coalition on Women and AIDS, 20, avenue Appia, CH-1211 Geneva 27, Switzerland, tel: +41.22.791.5412, fax: +41.22.791.4187, email: womenandaids@unaids.org, website: http://womenandaids.unaids.org/default.html, resources page: http://womenandaids.unaids.org/resources/default.html

The Global Coalition on Women and AIDS (GCWA) is a worldwide alliance of civil-society groups, networks of women with HIV and AIDS, governments, and UN organisations. The Coalition works at global, regional, and national levels to highlight the impact of AIDS on women and girls and mobilise actions to enable them to protect themselves from HIV and receive the care and support they need. The Coalition's resources page includes background papers from the Coalition on preventing HIV infection in girls and young women; violence against women and AIDS; securing women's property and inheritance rights; AIDS treatment; AIDS and girls' education; care, women, and AIDS; and microbicides, women, and AIDS. It also includes speeches from members of the Coalition, as well as links to relevant publications by other organisations.

GNP+ The Global Network of People Living with HIV/AIDS, P.O. Box 11726, 1001 GS Amsterdam, The Netherlands, tel: +31 20 423 4114, fax: +31 20 423 4224, email: infognp@gnpplus.net, website: www.gnpplus.net, library: www.gnpplus.net/component/option,com_docman/Itemid,53/

GNP+ works to improve the quality of life for all people living with HIV through advocating increased access to treatment, care, and prevention programmes, a decrease in the stigma and discrimination directed towards people living with HIV, and increased and more meaningful involvement of people living with HIV. Programme work centres on sexual and reproductive health and rights, human rights, and empowering people who live with HIV. Reports and dossiers can be downloaded from their website.

The International Community of Women living with HIV/AIDS (ICW), Main Office: Unit 6, Building 1, Canonbury Yard, 190a New North Road, London, N1 7BJ, UK, tel: +44 20 7704 0606, fax: +44 20 7704 8070, email: info@icw.org, website: www.icw.org, (the website provides contact details for regional contacts), publications page: www.icw.org/publications

ICW is a global network run by and for HIV-positive women. The network has nearly 4,000 members in over 90 countries, and uses English, French, and Spanish as its main working languages. The aim is to improve the situation of women living with HIV through self-empowerment and the exchange of information. While ICW membership is open to HIV-positive women only, the network has also started a care-givers' group, which is intended as a support network for women who may themselves be negative, untested, or HIV-positive, who are caring for others with HIV. Many useful publications including fact sheets, research papers, and personal testimonies from women affected by HIV can be downloaded from the organisation's publications page. In particular, the organisation makes a point of publishing research undertaken by HIV-positive women.

The International HIV/AIDS Alliance, International Secretariat: Queensberry House, 104–106 Queens Road, Brighton BN1 3XF, United Kingdom, tel: +44 (0)1273 718900, fax: +44 (0)1273 718901, email: mail@aidsalliance.org, website: www.aidsalliance.org

The Alliance is the European Union's largest HIV/AIDS-focused development organisation. Established in 1993, their work focuses on mobilising and strengthening communities so that they can respond to HIV themselves. Information on regional contacts can be found on their website, which also has links to a large selection of publications. These include many on gender and sexuality.

International Partnership for Microbicides, 8401 Colesville Road, Suite 200, Silver Spring, MD 20910, tel: +1 301-608-2221, fax: +1 301-608-2241, website: www.ipm-microbicides.org/index.htm

The International Partnership for Microbicides (IPM) is a non-profit product-development partnership (PDP) established in 2002. Its aim is to accelerate the development and availability of a safe and effective microbicide for use by women in developing countries as protection from HIV infection, by funding and/or initiating medical research. The IPM website provides information on microbicides, details of ongoing research projects, and access to a range of publications including fact sheets, policy papers, and academic articles.

International Women's Health Coalition, 333 Seventh Avenue, 6th floor, New York, NY 10001, USA, tel: +1 212 979 8500, fax: +1 212 979 9009, email: info@iwhc.org, website: www.iwhc.org, resource library on HIV/AIDS and other sexually transmitted infections: www.iwhc.org/resources/resources.cfm?classificationItemID=26

The International Women's Health Coalition promotes and protects the health and rights of women worldwide, with a particular focus on sexual and reproductive rights. This is achieved through advocacy and supporting women's-rights organisations throughout the world. The resource library features a wide range of different materials on women and HIV and other sexually transmitted infections. These include fact sheets, transcripts of speeches and panel discussions, and training materials. The website also provides links to other issues relevant to gender, health, and sexuality.

The UK Consortium on AIDS and International Development, Grayston Centre, 28 Charles Square, London N1 6HT, United Kingdom, tel: +44 (0)207 7324 4780, email: info@aidsconsortium.org.uk, website: www.aidsconsortium.org.uk

This consortium brings together over 80 organisations working to understand and develop effective approaches to the problems created by the HIV epidemic in developing countries. Principal activities include information exchange, networking, advocacy, and campaigning. The consortium has a working group dedicated to gender and HIV, and also publishes material on a wide range of issues. These can be downloaded from the website.

United Nations Development Fund for Women (UNIFEM), 304 East, 45th Street, 15th flr., New York, NY 10017 USA, website: www.unifem.org

UNIFEM is the women's fund at the United Nations. It provides financial and technical assistance to innovative programmes and strategies to foster women's empowerment and gender equality. Reversing the spread of HIV among women and girls is one of UNIFEM's core strategic activities.

UNAIDS, 20, Avenue Appia, CH-1211 Geneva 27, Switzerland, website: www.unaids.org, publications page: www.unaids.org/DocOrder/OrderForm.aspx

The Joint United Nations Programme on HIV/AIDS (UNAIDS) is one of the main advocates for accelerated, comprehensive, and co-ordinated global action on the epidemic. UNAIDS's mission is to lead, strengthen, and support an expanded response to HIV and AIDS that includes preventing transmission of HIV, providing care and support to those already living with the virus, reducing the vulnerability of individuals and communities to HIV, and alleviating the impact of the epidemic. An enormous selection of case studies, best-practice guidelines, research reports, and fact sheets can be downloaded from their publications page.

The United Nations Population Fund (UNFPA), 220 East 42nd Street, New York, NY 10017 USA, tel: +1 212-297-5000, website: www.unfpa.org

UNFPA is an international development agency that promotes the right of every woman, man, and child to enjoy a life of health and equal opportunity. One if its overarching goals is to prevent HIV.

Index

'n' shows material in notes

care *see* health care; support services
Chikankata 129
child-bearing 44, 94–5
    see also mothers; sexual and repro-
      ductive rights
child mortality, Africa 37
children xx, 9–11, 12
    African women in UK 93, 94–5, 98
    prevention and treatment 10
    stigmatisation 13
    Zimbabwe 9, 11, 14–16
    see also boys; Convention on the
      Rights of the Child (CRC); educa-
      tion; girls; orphans; young people
children's rights xx, 10, 13, 16–17
China 33, 35, 36
circumcision 163, 173*n*
coloured communities
    South Africa 21, 29–30*n*
    see also Atlantis
'Committed to youth' project 83–4
condom use 48, 50–51
    armed forces personnel 191
    Asia-Pacific region 34, 36
    Australia 82
    Bangladesh 33, 36
    Cambodia 61, 63, 67
    Côte d'Ivoire 49
    effectiveness 185
    India 34, 48, 81
    married couples xviii, 46
    promotion of 39, 82, 88, 130, 174*n*
    Stepping Stones training package
      128, 129
    Thailand 45–6, 48
    Uganda 50–1, 128
    women 48, 52, 128, 153
    young men 26, 27, 29, 77, 79, 82, 88
    young men's attitudes to 76, 77, 78,
      81, 82
    Zimbabwe 126
    see also female condoms; safe sex
consultation *see* stakeholder involvement
    consumerism 169–70
contraception 46–9, 50–1, 52, 76–7, 128, 153
    see also condom use; family planning
Convention on the Elimination of All
    Forms of Discrimination Against
    Women (CEDAW) xx, 10–11, 15, 157
Convention on the Rights of the Child
    (CRC) xx, 10, 15, 16
CORO for Literacy 81
Côte d'Ivoire 49
credit and loans
    rural communities 105, 108, 114–5, 118

    see also household finances
criminalisation 157

Denmark 82
Department for International
    Development (DFID), United Kingdom
    132–3
depression *see* mental health
disclosure of HIV status 97–9, 116, 154,
    157
discordant relationships 153, 161*n*, 174*n*
drug trials 168
drug users 32–3, 36, 163, 167
drugs *see* treatment

Eastern Europe xxii, 5, 167
    see also Estonia; Romania
education
    African women in UK 92–3
    children 10
    Estonia 80
    girls 11–12, 15, 16, 17, 107–8, 164
    India 81–2
    Kenya 177
    mothers 107–8
    orphans 12, 107–8, 113
    Papua New Guinea 139
    positive living 116
    prevalence rates and 39
    staffing xiv
    sub-Saharan Africa 107–8, 113
    Thailand 70
    traditional healers 130
    Uganda 113, 130
    women and 151, 164
    young men 81–2, 86, 87
    Zimbabwe 15, 16, 39, 126
    see also training
employment xiv, 13, 16, 34–5, 93, 139,
    141–3
Estonia 80
Europe xxi, 5, 37, 50, 54*n*
    see also Belgium; Eastern Europe;
      Netherlands; United Kingdom

faith-based organisations 169
Family Health International (FHI) 62, 63
family planning 46–7, 49, 52–3, 174*n*
    see also contraception; Gambian
      Family Planning Association;
      International Planned Parenthood
      Federation (IPPF); Planned
      Parenthood Association of South
      Africa; Swedish Family Planning
      Association (RFSU)

farm schools see agriculture; Kitovu Mobile Farm School Project

Farmer Field Schools for Organic Cotton Production Project 107, 111

fathers, young men xxii, 86

female condoms 48, 82, 164, 165

feminism 5–6, 8, 69, 72n

fertility

women xxi, 49–51

see also child-bearing; contraception

finances see household finances

food 38, 111, 116

see also agriculture

France, African women immigrants 49

Gambia 128, 129, 134n

Gambian Family Planning Association 128

gangsterism, South Africa 20–31

gatekeepers 86, 117, 127, 134

gay men 5, 62, 69–70, 82–4, 162–3

see also kathoey

men who have sex with men

gender-based violence xiv–xv

Brazil 79, 127–8

gangsterism and 23

girls 15

Papua New Guinea xxii–xxiii, 137

Stepping Stones training package 129

young men xx, 79, 80, 127–8

see also sexual violence; violence against women

gender equality/inequality xiv, xv, 71

Asia-Pacific region 33–5, 41

family planning 46

HIV and AIDS impact on livelihoods 38

men's and boys' involvement in combatting xv, 77–8, 86, 127

national and international organisations 150, 155, 169

Papua New Guinea 137–46

South Africa 158

Swaziland 158

Zimbabwe 126

Gender Equitable Men Scale 79, 91n

gender identities xxi, xxiii, 61–74, 81

see also masculinity; transgender identities

gender mainstreaming 40, 138, 143–4

girls 9–18

Africa 5, 12, 13–14

Asia-Pacific region 33

education 11–12, 15, 16, 17, 107–8, 164

poverty 13–14

sub-Saharan Africa xx, 5, 107–8, 166

support for xiv, 17–18

survival sex 5

treatment and prevention xiv

violence 33

Zimbabwe xx, 12, 13–14, 15–17

see also young women

Global Fund to fight AIDS, Tuberculosis and Malaria (GFATM) xiv, xxvn, 138

Global Network of People living with HIV (GNP+) 86, 163

globalisation xix–xx, 3–5, 61, 70, 168–9

governance 36–7, 39, 40–1

health care 165–6

African women in UK 99–100

Asia 34

children 10, 12

Papua New Guinea 139

South Africa 158

staff xiv, 119

Swaziland 156

women 151, 155, 156

Zimbabwe 126

see also sexual and reproductive health (SRH); traditional healers; treatment

Holland see Netherlands

homophobia xiii, xxii, 80, 162, 163, 169

homosexuals see gay men; men who have sex with men

horticultural training 111

household finances

African women immigrants 95–6

Asia-Pacific region 34–5, 37–8

effect of Stepping Stones training package 129

Papua New Guinea 141–2

rural communities 105, 108, 110, 111, 112–3

Zimbabwe 126

see also credit and loans; transactional sex

human rights xix, xx, 5, 16–17, 168

see also children's rights

Humsafar Trust 41

immigrants xxii, 49, 92–101

incomes see household finances

India

condom use 34, 48, 81

drug users 36

education 81–2

masculinity 81

men who have sex with men 41, 83

prevalence rates 32, 33, 34, 35–6, 134n

mental health 97–8, 170
Mexico 85
microbicides 48, 155, 164–5
migration 35, 119, 137, 139–40, 169
    see also African women immigrants
military forces 158
mobility see migration
mortality rates
    Papua New Guinea 139
    see also infant mortality; life expectancy
mothers 94–5, 154
    drug users 167
    education 107–8
    Papua New Guinea 139
    reproductive choice xx–xxi, 44–57
    sub-Saharan Africa 107–8
    Uganda 115
    see also child-bearing; pregnant
        women; sexual and reproductive
        rights; women
Movement of Men Against AIDS in
    Kenya (MMAAK) 86, 173n
Mpowerment project 83
multi-sectoral approaches 117–8, 134
Musasa Project 131, 135n
Myanmar
    drug users 167
    see also Burma

National Audit 41
National Community of Women Living
    with AIDS in Uganda 107, 113–4
Natural Resources Institute (NRI) 106–7
NAZ foundation 83
'negative income shock' 38
Nepal xxii, 125, 126, 131
Netherlands 82
Nicaragua xxii, 80
Nigeria 132
Nigerian women in UK 98, 99, 100
North America 54n, 68
    see also United States
nutrition see food

Oil Palm Industry Corporation (OPIC)
    140, 141, 143
Oil Palm Research Agency (OPRA) 143
orphans 12–13
    Africa 5
    education 12, 107–8, 113
    migration 119
    property rights 13, 113
    'small house' phenomenon 14
    sub-Saharan Africa 105, 107–8, 111,
        113, 114–5, 117, 118

Tanzania 113
Uganda 112, 113
women's role in providing for 151
Zimbabwe 9–10, 11, 13, 15–16

Pakistan xxii, 36, 132–3
Papua New Guinea xxii–xxiii, 137–46
participation see stakeholder involvement
People with AIDS Development
    Association 107
pharmaceutical companies 168
Planned Parenthood Association of South
    Africa 128
POLICY project 153, 157, 158, 161n
positive living 116
positive prevention 84, 91n
poverty 6, 13–14, 119, 126, 137
pregnant women xxvn, 7, 45, 54n, 155,
    156, 165–6
    see also mothers
President's Emergency Programme for
    AIDS Relief (PEPFAR) xiv
prevention
    HIV and AIDS xiv, 10, 29, 45, 164
    see also condom use; microbicides;
        positive prevention; safe sex
Promundo 81, 127–8
property rights
    orphans 13, 113
    Stepping Stones training package 129
    women and girls 13, 17, 105, 126,
        140, 166–7
Pros saat ('short hairs') 62–3, 66, 69, 70
prostitution see sex workers

rape xxvn, 65, 93, 131, 139, 140
    see also sexual violence
'real men'
    Cambodia 64, 65, 70
    see also masculinity
religious organisations 169
reproductive health see sexual and repro-
    ductive health (SRH)
Reproductive Health Alliance 159
reproductive rights see sexual and repro-
    ductive rights
Romania 85
rural communities xxii, 105–122, 128–9,
    155
Russia xxi

safe sex
    Asia-Pacific region 34, 36
    Cambodia 63, 67
    gay men 83–4

young men 36, 76, 81–2
  Zambia 52
  see also condom use
Sak klay ('short hairs') 62–3, 66, 69, 70
same-sex relationships 62, 68, 70
  see also gay men; men who have sex
    with men
Senegal 37
seroconcordant relationships 85, 92*n*
seropositive young people 84–5, 91*n*
sex work 61
  see also survival sex; transactional sex
sex workers
  Asia 35–6
  Bangladesh 33, 141
  blamed for HIV transmission 45
  Bradford xxii, 124, 125, 126, 131
  Burma 33
  Cambodia 61, 62, 63, 64, 65, 67, 68
  drug users 167
  girls in Africa 5, 12, 13–14
  India 141
  Nepal xxii, 125, 126, 131
  Pakistan 36
  Shakti Sex Worker Projects 141
  Thailand 45–6
  violence xxii, 124, 125
sexual and reproductive health (SRH)
  Asia-Pacific region 34
  Swaziland 158
  young men 76, 77, 78, 80, 84–5, 87–9
  see also health care
sexual and reproductive rights 165–6
  men xxii, 163
  women xx–xxi, xxiii, 44–57, 153, 154,
    157–8
sexual violence 26–7, 28, 139
  see also gender-based violence; rape
sexually transmitted infections
  Brazil 79
  HIV and AIDS and 39
  Papua New Guinea 139, 140
  United Kingdom xvi
Shakti Sex Worker Projects 141
'short hairs' 62–3, 66, 69, 70
'small house' phenomenon 14
South Africa
  advocacy training 150, 152–6
  Asia-Pacific region compared to 38
  coloured communities 21, 29–30*n*
  condom use 26, 27, 29
  criminalisation 157
  gangsterism 20–31
  gender equality/inequality 158
  health care 158

Khayelitsha 25–6
  male life expectancy 21
  marriage 158
  masculinity 23, 25, 26–7
  microfinance 141, 142
  Stepping Stones training package
    128–9
  Treatment Action Campaign (TAC) 7
  Womandla 158–9
  women 5, 157–9
  young men xx, 20–31
South African Medical Research Council
  128, 190
Southern Africa xx, xxiii, 3–5, 159
Southern African AIDS Trust (SAT) 16
Srei Sros ('long hairs') 63–5, 66, 67, 69,
  70–1, 72*n*
stakeholder involvement xxii, 133, 170
  International Community of Women
    Living with HIV (ICW) 168
  men xv, xxii
  research 167–8
  rural communities 107, 117
  women xiv, 149–61
  see also advocacy; Working Women's
    Project
Stepping Stones training package 128–9,
  134–5*n*
stigmatisation
  Africa 154, 157
  African women immigrants in UK
    97–8
  children 13
  men 163
  men who have sex with men 83
  rural communities in sub-Saharan
    Africa 108, 115, 116, 117, 118
  women 154, 157, 163
  Zambia 184
  Zimbabwe 126
sub-Saharan Africa
  girls xx, 5, 107–8, 166
  property rights 166
  rural communities xxii, 105–122,
    128–9
  statistics 32, 37, 105
  Stepping Stones training package
    128–9
  women xx, 92
    agricultural training 111
    credit and loans 114–5
    poverty 119
    property rights 166
    rural communities 108, 111, 114–5,
    119

www.ingramcontent.com/pod-product-compliance
Lightning Source LLC
Chambersburg PA
CBHW072105040426
42334CB00042B/2346